the
Healthy Pregnancy
Journal

The Sears Parenting Library

The Healthy Pregnancy Book

The Baby Book

The Birth Book

The Breastfeeding Book

The Baby Sleep Book

The Attachment Parenting Book

The Portable Pediatrician

The Fussy Baby Book

The Family Nutrition Book

The Premature Baby Book

Also by Martha and Hayden Sears

25 Things Every New Mom Should Know:
Essential First Steps for Mothers

25 Things Every New Dad Should Know:
Essential First Steps for Fathers

the Healthy Pregnancy Journal

A Weekly Guide for Reflecting on
Your Pregnancy and Preparing Your Heart,
Body, and Mind for Motherhood

MARTHA SEARS, RN
HAYDEN SEARS, MA

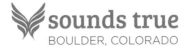

sounds true
BOULDER, COLORADO

Sounds True
Boulder, CO 80306

Published 2019

Cover design by Jennifer Miles
Book design by Beth Skelley
Interior art by Jennifer Miles

Printed in Canada

ISBN: 978-1-68364-247-3

10 9 8 7 6 5 4 3 2 1

Contents

Your Journey into Motherhood

Our pregnancies were some of the most special times in our lives, and though the days seemed long, the months flew by. By the time your baby arrives, we imagine you'll agree with us.

So many emotional and physical changes happen—seemingly all at once. We remember feeling both empowered and vulnerable, beautiful and dumpy, and like superheroes and scaredy-cats. But looking back now, it is sometimes difficult to recall specific memories from our own pregnancy journeys (Martha: 7 and Hayden: 3).

We developed *The Healthy Pregnancy Journal* as a guide to help you reflect on this most special time, to work through the beautiful chaos of pregnancy by journaling, to keep you on track to having a healthy pregnancy, and to create a keepsake that you can return to in years to come. Throughout the journal, we call on our experience as health, childbirth, breastfeeding and parenting educators to help you bond with your baby before birth and offer important advice to keep you and your baby thriving during pregnancy. It is the perfect companion to *The Healthy Pregnancy Book: Everything You Need to Know from America's Baby Experts*, part of the Sears Parenting Library.

Our hope is that this journal will help you connect with yourself and your baby on a deeper level—one of our favorite parts of the journal is where you write a monthly love letter to your growing child. You may want to share this with your child one day! But in our minds, a journal equally embraces the happy, cute moments, like bump pics, baby showers, and first kicks, and the parts of pregnancy that aren't as shareable—the fears, the worries, and the meltdowns. That is why we also provide insightful and often intimate prompts to encourage you to write down your innermost thoughts, whether those thoughts are fit for public consumption or not. We want to create a space for all your feelings and experiences as you prepare to be a mom, whether it's for the first or the fourth time.

The sweet spot of pregnancy gives way, oh so quickly, to the whole new world of motherhood. *The Healthy Pregnancy Journal* opens up the space for you to reflect on your mental, emotional, and physical evolution over the course of pregnancy and to embrace each phase for what it adds to your life. We look forward to guiding you on this momentous and spectacular journey.

With love,
Martha and Hayden

This Journal

While it is common to think of pregnancy as being 9 months, the modern way of counting the beginning of pregnancy from the first missed period makes it 40 weeks or approximately 10 months long. Therefore, this journal also begins on the first day of your last period. Even though you may not have this journal at the beginning of your pregnancy, it is valuable to go back and start it at the beginning to reflect on and memorialize your pre-baby life and those early days.

Each week is centered around a theme, for example, changes to your physical body, shifting relationships, pregnancy milestones, and planning for birth. That said, every pregnancy journey is different, and if a certain theme doesn't match where you're at, come back to it when it feels right for you. This is your chronicle of your pregnancy—use the journal as it serves your needs. Also included in each week are information around the development of your baby, space for photos, and a "Pro-Pregnancy Tip" to help you manage the changes that pregnancy brings.

At the end of each month, we provide open space to record your hopes and dreams in a way that resonates with you—words, drawings, quotes, or even magazine clippings. Think of it as your monthly vision board. We also include a page for you to talk directly to your baby, a love note that you can pass on to your child in the years to come—perhaps when he or she becomes a parent.

The end of the journal is dedicated to chronicling the birth of your baby, including vital statistics, pictures, your birth story, and your own sweet words to the newest love in your life.

The journaling will begin soon, in just a few pages. But we hope you will first start with the "Healthy Pregnancy Dos and Don'ts" on the pages that follow, and refer back to them as needed. For a list of our favorite pregnancy and parenting-related tools and resources, refer to the back of the journal.

Dos and Don'ts

Everyone you ask (including your health-care provider) will have a specific list of pregnancy dos and don'ts, and some of them may even conflict. It is easy to get overwhelmed when you have information coming at you from all sides and the stakes seem so high. Here's a quick guide to the changes health-care providers and pregnancy coaches agree you should make to your life and environment for a healthy pregnancy, perhaps the most important one being: Don't stress, Mama. You got this!

Healthy Pregnancy Nutrition

One of the first worries that comes up for pregnant women is whether what they're eating is safe and nourishing for Baby. In truth, your healthy pregnancy eating should be quite similar to normal healthy eating—with just a few tweaks.

Eat and Drink

It is important to remember that pregnant women need only 100 extra calories per day in the first trimester, and between 300 and 500 daily in the second and third trimesters. Drink at least eight (ideally 10) glasses of filtered water daily. Eat organic whenever you can, but especially the fruits and veggies known to have high levels of pesticides (also known as the Dirty Dozen): celery, peaches, strawberries, apples, blueberries, nectarines, bell peppers, spinach, cherries, kale and collard greens, potatoes, and grapes.

Eat organic whenever you can, especially the Dirty Dozen.

Focus on the quality of your food more than the quantity. These are the top nutrient-dense foods:

- fish (Visit AskDrSears.com to read about safe seafood.)
- nuts, raw are best
- greens
- avocados
- eggs
- plain Greek yogurt
- blueberries
- beans and lentils
- flaxseeds and flax meal
- extra-virgin olive oil
- tofu
- oatmeal

Supplements

While supplements can't take the place of balanced nutrition, they can be helpful to ensure you are getting enough of the most important nutrients necessary to grow a healthy baby—especially if you're suffering from food aversions and nausea.

- Take nutritional supplements and find food sources that include:

  1. folic acid or folate (RDA: 600 mcg) in the form of methyl folate if possible

2. omega-3s (RDA: 1,000 mg)

3. iron (RDA: 30 mg), supplement only
   if your iron level is low

- Take a vitamin D3 supplement if your
  vitamin D levels are low.

- Take a probiotic for gut health.

- Talk to your health-care provider about any prescription
  or over-the-counter medication you are taking
  to ensure it is safe to use during pregnancy.

- We recommend using a fruit and vegetable
  supplement to get extra nutrients from whole
  food (our favorite is Juice Plus+).

Avoid and Limit

- Avoid illegal drugs.

- Avoid alcohol and marijuana.

- Avoid high-mercury fish like swordfish and shark.

- Avoid unpasteurized foods, deli meats
  containing nitrites, and soft cheeses.

- Limit caffeine to the equivalent of
  about 1 cup of coffee a day.

- Limit highly processed foods and beverages and
  those containing artificial dyes and sweeteners.

Limit caffeine
to about 1 cup of
coffee a day.

Healthy Pregnancy Exercise

Even for pregnant women, the rule still stands: the more you move, the healthier you are. However, the most important thing is to lean into what your body is feeling. If you're tired, rest. When you feel ready, be sure to consult your health-care provider before embarking on a new-to-you exercise program.

- Start with familiar activities.

- Keep your heart rate below 140 beats per minute.

- Don't push too hard: if you experience dizziness, headaches, or shortness of breath, stop.

- Avoid lying on your back after the fourth month.

- Practice your Kegel exercises to tone your pelvic floor.

Avoid lying on your back after the fourth month.

Healthy Pregnancy Lifestyle and Environment

It is no coincidence that a pregnant woman is most sensitive to environmental smells and toxins at the time when her baby is most vulnerable to them: the first trimester. Once you find out you are pregnant, here's what to do to keep your environment safe for you and your baby.

- If you smoke or vape, quit. Also, stay away from places and people who smoke to avoid second- and thirdhand exposure.

- Drink filtered water.

- Consider investing in a HEPA air filter or purifier for your home.

- Stock your home with BPA-free bottles and containers.

- Avoid aerosol cleaners and beauty products that contain volatile organic compounds (VOCs).

- Don't change cat litter boxes (get your partner, close family, or friends to do it for you).

- Only go to well-ventilated beauty salons.

- Use a sunscreen with an SPF factor of at least 30 daily.

- Work on getting at least seven hours of sleep a day—including naps.

- Explore how you can practice self-care to mellow your mind, soothe your spirit, and relax your body (for example, meditation, massage, nature walks, and warm baths).

- Surround yourself with people who support you and lift you up.

- Be kind to yourself.

Being healthy is a journey without an end destination, and it is important to remember that what is good and healthy for you will be good and healthy for your baby. Do the best that you can on any given day and trust that Baby is growing just as he or she should.

Only go to well-ventilated beauty salons.

YOUR HEALTHY
Pregnancy Goals

Based on the dos and don'ts you just read, what are the top changes you want to make to your life and environment while pregnant? Try focusing on a goal or two each month and use the prompts throughout the journal to evaluate your progress and any shifts you may need to make.

Set yourself up for success by setting goals that are specific, measurable, and attainable. Remember, it can take upwards of 21 days to create a new habit if you can stick to it on a daily basis.

That said, this process is meant to serve you on your journey, not be a source of guilt or embarrassment. Make your goals realistic for where you are in your life and celebrate your achievements. Don't get bogged down on what you don't accomplish.

Nutrition Goals

1 _____

_____

2 _____

_____

3 _____

_____

Exercise and Activity Goals

1 _____

_____

2 _____

_____

3 _____

_____

Lifestyle and Environment Goals

1 _____

_____

2 _____

_____

3 _____

_____

Take a Deep Breath

Weeks 1 Through 4

Congratulations on your pregnancy! If you weren't before, now you are a mother. Be prepared to be amazed at what your body will accomplish over the next 40 weeks.

Staying in the moment, especially with all the excitement and, let's face it, anxiety that comes with a new pregnancy can be difficult. But whether this is your first baby or your fourth, it is important to bear witness to all the changes going on in your body and around you as you nurture this new life.

The conventional way to start counting your pregnancy is from the first day of your last menstrual period—about two weeks before sperm meets egg. Most women aren't aware that they are pregnant until at least week 4 and often later. If that's your case, come back to this month and record in retrospect what you were thinking and feeling at the start of this amazing life journey you may not have even known you were on!

What Baby Wants You to Know

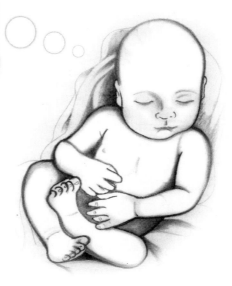

I'm so excited to start this journey with you!

Happy, healthy moms are the most likely to have happy, healthy babies! Now is the time to begin creating habits around the goals you set for yourself in the last section.

Staying calm and managing your stress helps to create a soothing and healthy environment for me to grow.

Listen to your body. For example, if you begin to have intense food cravings, find the healthiest version of that food and eat up!

Pre-Pregnancy Pic!

Date _____

Who took this picture? _____

What do I love about it? _____

Where was I? _____

How old was I then? _____

What was on my mind? _____

How was I feeling? _____

What do I want to remember about this day and this time in my life? _____

_____

Health Check-In

Am I getting enough sleep (at least seven hours)?

Am I staying hydrated (drinking eight or more glasses of water daily)?

Am I managing my stress?

How?

Am I exercising regularly and safely?

How am I doing on my healthy pregnancy goals?

Martha's Pregnancy Salad

This superfood salad is the perfect pregnancy meal.
Customize it with your own favorites.

Salad

1	4-ounce grilled or canned salmon filet
4	ounces kidney beans
3	cups spinach
¼	cup chopped tomatoes
1	tablespoon raw sunflower or sesame seeds
1	egg, hard-boiled and sliced

Dressing

1	tablespoon extra virgin olive oil
	juice of half a lemon or lime
½	teaspoon turmeric
	black pepper and salt, to taste

Directions

Mix the dressing ingredients together then combine salad ingredients, lightly toss with the dressing, and top with salmon.

Notes

WEEK 1 Who Am I?

No baby on board, yet. If your tummy is feeling a bit larger than usual, chalk it up to menstrual bloat.

How would I describe myself as a woman?
What are my talents and skills?

_____

_____

_____

_____

_____

What do I like most about my pre-baby body?

_____

_____

_____

_____

_____

Life as you know it is about to change!

Week 1 begins on the first day of your last period, before you actually get pregnant. Fertilization and implantation don't happen until weeks 2 and 3.

What does a typical day in my life look like?
What are my favorite activities?

_____

_____

_____

_____

What was my pre-baby life plan?

_____

_____

_____

_____

What do I like most about my pre-baby life?

_____

_____

_____

_____

WEEK 2   My Community

Common ovulation signs include thin, clear, stringy cervical mucus, pelvic ache, breast tenderness, and increased sex drive. Which did you experience (if any)?

So much love
is coming
your way!

Before I Was Pregnant . . .

What was going on in my family and relationships?

_____

_____

_____

_____

Toward the end
of week 2, your
body is likely
getting ready
to ovulate.

What was going on in the world?

_____

_____

_____

_____

Which of my closest friends and family already have kids?

_____

_____

_____

_____

How do I feel about other people's kids?

_____

_____

_____

_____

_____

Who are the babies in my life that I feel most connected to?

_____

_____

_____

_____

_____

What do I like most about babies?

_____

_____

_____

_____

_____

Pro-Pregnancy Tip

Pregnancy can be isolating. Joining a pregnancy group with women due around the same time as you is a great way to find community and expand your village. You can often find out about pregnancy groups to join through your hospital or birthing center, your health-care provider, or local baby stores. Examples include prenatal yoga, water aerobics, and meet-up groups.

WEEK 3 Getting Pregnant

This is the week you likely conceived. Can you pinpoint the occasion?

When and where do I think I conceived?

_____

_____

_____

_____

What were my thoughts on the idea of getting pregnant? Was my age a factor?

_____

_____

_____

_____

How did I find out I was pregnant? Where was I?

_____

_____

_____

_____

You don't know it yet, but I'm here!

Even before you emotionally feel or physically look pregnant, a lot is going on inside of you. First comes fertilization (sperm meets egg), then implantation, when Baby finds a comfortable nest in the plush lining of your uterus.

How did I tell my partner?

_____

_____

_____

_____

_____

_____

_____

Who were the first three people I told, and what were
their reactions?

_____

_____

_____

_____

_____

_____

_____

Pro-Pregnancy Tip

Go for a "no-white"
diet during pregnancy.
Replace white bread
with whole grain
bread, regular spuds
with sweet potatoes,
and white rice with
brown or wild rice.
Refined white foods
tend to be stripped
of their nutrients, so
make each bite you
take more valuable
to you and Baby by
saying no to white.
The more colorful your
plate, the more likely it
is to contain the wide
range of vitamins and
minerals it takes to
grow a healthy baby.

WEEK 4 Becoming a Mom

Feeling tired? The overwhelming fatigue many newly pregnant women come to experience is your body and your brain urging you to tune in to your and your baby's needs. At this stage, rest is one of the best ways to nurture your growing baby.

What were my initial thoughts, feelings, and reactions when I saw the positive pregnancy test?

_____

_____

_____

_____

_____

I've already multiplied into the millions of cells that will form all my organs!

Did I always want kids?

_____

_____

_____

_____

_____

_____

This week is usually marked by a missed period. What was your experience?

What do I admire most about my own mother and other mothers in my life?

_____

_____

_____

_____

Describe the mother you want to be:

_____

_____

_____

_____

What do I think being a mom will be like for me?

_____

_____

_____

_____

Pro-Pregnancy Tip

For many newly pregnant women, a hypersensitivity to odors is the first clue that a bun is in the oven. Does your dog all of a sudden smell more "doggy"? Can you smell someone's perfume or cologne from across the room?

Month 1 Closing Thoughts
and Final Reflections

What am I most excited about?

_____

_____

_____

_____

What are my worries or fears?

_____

_____

_____

_____

What memories will I treasure from this month?

_____

_____

_____

_____

My Thoughts, Dreams, and Hopes

Use this free space to doodle, record your dreams and other random musings, or capture images, quotes, and clippings that reflect what you are feeling and focused on related to your pregnancy this month.

A Love Note (or Poem) to My Growing Baby

Dear Baby,

_____

_____

_____

_____

_____

_____

_____

_____

_____

_____

_____

_____

_____

_____

Picture of a Special Moment from Month 1!

Date _____

Who took this picture? _____

Where was I? _____

What was on my mind? _____

_____

How was I feeling? _____

_____

What do I want to remember about this day? _____

_____

Feeling Pregnant

Weeks 5 Through 8

What does it feel like to have a new life growing inside you? While you may not have even known you were pregnant in month 1, month 2 is a totally different story. Your body is working hard to grow your baby, and it likely isn't being shy in letting you know. Hopefully, excitement will help you to take all these changes in stride, but if that's not always the case, don't stress. Pregnancy is filled with lots of ups and downs for every woman.

I'm teeny tiny!

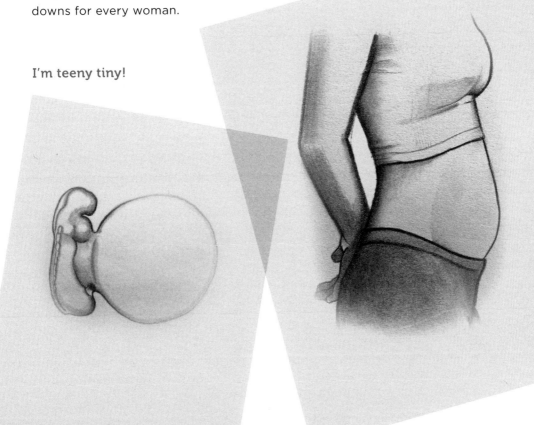

What Baby Wants You to Know

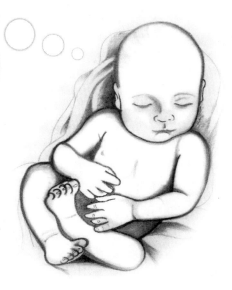

When you take
care of you,
you are taking
care of me, Mama.

If food isn't your friend right now, a prenatal supplement is a great way to ensure I get all the nutrients I need to grow big and strong.

Sleep! It takes a lot of energy to grow a new human, and at least when you're sleeping, you're not nauseated.

Check your skin and beauty products to make sure they are baby-safe. Avoid using ones that contain phthalates, retinols, and salicylic acid.

Pro-Pregnancy Tips
to Ease Early-Pregnancy Discomforts

Common pregnancy symptoms during this month include extreme fatigue, nausea, frequent urination, and feeling like you're on an emotional rollercoaster—all before your baby is even the size of a peanut! Here are our tried-and-true tips for comforting your body, mind, and soul.

1. **Explore acupressure.** There's an acupressure point about two inches above your wrist that is said to relieve nausea and vomiting. Try pressing it yourself or purchase some acupressure bands to stimulate this magical pressure point.

2. **Aim for small, frequent meals.** If you are able to keep food down, graze on small, nutrient-dense, and easily digestible meals like soups and smoothies throughout the day. Try keeping some salty crackers or rice cakes by your bed to nibble on as soon as you wake to ease early morning nausea.

3. **Position yourself for optimal digestion.** You can prevent or at least minimize heartburn by staying upright for at least a half hour after meals and sleeping on your left side.

4. **Avoid common morning sickness triggers.** The most common offenders include body odors, stale or leftover food in the fridge, coffee, gasoline, solvent fumes, garbage, scented cosmetics and toiletries, and pungent aromas of cooking foods.

5. **Go for a walk.** A change of environment and a breath of fresh air will help you get your mind off your discomforts, energize your body, and soothe your worries.

6. **Take it easy—and delegate.** It's totally understandable why even thinking about your normal list of to-dos suddenly feels so

exhausting—a great deal of your energy has now been redirected toward supporting a new life. Do only what you feel you must and recruit your partner, friends, and family to help you with the rest. Anything that you can do to alleviate stress will help you feel more comfortable.

7. **Sleep it off.** It is fortunate that the extreme need for sleep coincides with the morning sickness phase. To the extent that you can, listen to your body, and rest as much and as often as you can.

8. **Use natural anti-nausea remedies.** Ginger and peppermint can naturally ease nausea. Try it in the form of tea, drinks, chews, and candy. The aroma of peppermint or freshly cut lemon can also help.

Bump (or No Bump) Pic!

Date _____

Who took this picture? _____

Where was I? _____

What was on my mind? _____

_____

How was I feeling? _____

_____

What do I want to remember about this day? _____

_____

Health Check-In

Am I getting enough sleep (at least seven hours)?

_____

_____

_____

Am I staying hydrated (drinking eight or more glasses of water daily)?

_____

_____

Am I managing my stress?

_____

How?

_____

_____

Am I exercising regularly and safely?

_____

How am I doing on my healthy pregnancy goals?

_____

_____

_____

Hayden's Pregnancy Super Smoothie

Don't have the time (or stomach) for solid food? Healthy smoothies are a great way to keep up your nutrition and are often easier on your digestive system. Just remember to sip slowly! Start with the recipe below and modify it to your taste and desired quantity. Add more liquid (water, vegetable juice, or nut milk) to get your preferred consistency. Add ice if not using frozen fruit.

2   handfuls kale or spinach

8   ounces liquid (water, coconut water, or almond milk)

1   cup low-fat or full-fat Greek yogurt

1   cup blueberries

1   banana or other fruit of your choice

2   tablespoons ground flaxseeds

1   teaspoon cinnamon

3   ounces firm tofu or 1 tablespoon almond butter (optional)

1   tablespoon blackstrap molasses or honey (optional)

1   scoop Juice Plus+ Complete protein powder

Directions

Blend all the above ingredients in a high-powered blender and sip.

Notes

WEEK 5 My Little Secret

This is a sacred moment in time as just you, and your inner circle, know about this monumental adventure beginning to unfold. Treasure this personal time before your whole world is invited in to be part of your experience.

Do you know I'm here yet?

Who suspected I was pregnant (even before I knew)?

_____

_____

_____

_____

Your baby may only be the size of a seed, but his or her presence is likely already starting to loom large in your everyday life!

When will I break the news I am expecting?

_____

_____

_____

_____

How do I feel about telling people?

_____

_____

_____

In what fun and unique ways can I let people know?

_____

_____

_____

Am I going to find out the sex of the baby?

_____

PROS	CONS

Am I hoping for a boy or a girl?

_____

_____

_____

What does my partner want?

_____

_____

_____

_____

WEEK 6
My Changing Body . . . and Life

I have a heart, and it's beating twice as fast as yours!

Ambivalence about being pregnant—even if the pregnancy was planned—is very common as your mind tries to keep up with the rapid changes in your body.

What in my life is going better than expected?
What is the hardest thing I'm dealing with?

_____

_____

_____

_____

_____

For most women, nausea peaks in month 2. Hormones are what causes nausea during pregnancy and are signs that your baby is growing normally, although that might not be much comfort when you're feeling like you're stuck on a little tugboat on the high seas.

When did nausea first hit? How did fatigue grab me?
Record any vivid memories or stories about those moments.

_____

_____

_____

_____

_____

In what ways have morning sickness, fatigue, and rollercoaster emotions been affecting my . . . (And what has helped?)

body

_____

_____

_____

_____

_____

mood

_____

_____

_____

_____

_____

relationships

_____

_____

_____

_____

_____

Pro-Pregnancy Tip

Recent studies on vitamin D have shown that a significant portion of pregnant women (and of the general population) are not getting enough of this critical vitamin. Deficiencies can be associated with increased C-section rates, more allergies in Baby, and weaker bones in Baby and Mom. Especially if you are a vegetarian, live in a cold climate, or have a dark complexion, you have an increased risk for low vitamin D. Talk to your health-care provider about getting tested. The two best sources are salmon and sunshine (about 15 minutes a day without sunscreen), and a vitamin D3 supplement is highly recommended.

WEEK 7 My Hopes and Fears

I have little buds for arms, legs, and fingers, and pits for developing eyes, ears, and a nose!

Having a support system in place for pregnancy and all that comes after can make the journey so much easier and enjoyable. Think about whom you can turn to when you are feeling nervous or fearful about the changes ahead.

I hope my baby has my . . .

_____

_____

_____

_____

_____

Feeling a bit like your adolescent self? Much like when you went through puberty, hormonal changes during pregnancy can cause sore, swollen breasts as well as throbbing or shooting sensations in your chest. In addition, your areolas may enlarge and darken, and your veins become more noticeable.

I hope my baby has my partner's . . .

_____

_____

_____

_____

_____

What are my greatest fears around pregnancy, birth,
and being a mom?

_____

_____

_____

_____

What are my feelings or fears about miscarrying?

Pro-Pregnancy Tip

The fear of miscarriage
is common in the first
trimester, especially
if it has happened
to you before or to
someone close to
you. If this fear seems
overwhelming, be
sure to talk with your
health-care provider.

_____

_____

_____

_____

What can I do to work through my pregnancy-related fears?

_____

_____

_____

_____

WEEK 8 Creating Space

If the slightest noises are putting you on edge and you feel like everyone is asking too much of you, focus on creating a peaceful space for you and your growing babe away from the irritations of everyday life—even if it's just for 10 minutes a day.

Where in my home can I create a peaceful space for calm reflection?

_____

_____

_____

_____

What do I want to change about my life before the baby comes?

_____

_____

_____

_____

What do I hope will stay the same?

_____

_____

_____

_____

Look Ma, I can move my budding arms and legs!

Less talked about early-pregnancy symptoms include increased saliva production and thirst—two good reasons to sip, sip, sip all day long (preferably water or a green smoothie).

What is my vision for Baby's nursery? (Include notes, pictures, and other inspiration in this blank space.)

Pro-Pregnancy Tip

What are the things about pregnancy and having a baby that you're most looking forward to? Designing a nursery? A big, round pregnant belly? Tiny baby shoes? Do something that sparks those good feelings—like shopping for nursery items, maternity clothes, or baby clothing—to keep your mind on all the amazing things in store for your journey.

Month 2 Closing Thoughts
and Final Reflections

What were my weirdest pregnancy symptoms?

What foods made me feel good?

What foods made me feel bad?

What progress did I make on my healthy pregnancy goals?
Do I need to add to or shift my goals in any way?

What are my favorite baby names so far?

NAME	ORIGIN AND MEANING

What memories will I treasure from this month?

My Thoughts, Dreams, and Hopes

Use this free space to sketch, record your dreams and other random musings, or capture images, quotes, and clippings that reflect what you are feeling and focused on related to your pregnancy this month.

A Love Note (or Poem) to My Growing Baby

Dear Baby,

Picture of a Special Moment from Month 2!

Date _____

Who took this picture? _____

Where was I? _____

What was on my mind? _____

_____

How was I feeling? _____

_____

What do I want to remember about this day? _____

_____

Almost Showing

Weeks 9 Through 12

The highlights of this month will likely offset the physical and emotional demands that have been so dominant for the past couple of months. For many women, the discomforts of the first trimester will start to ease up and energy levels begin to increase by the end of month 3. Your emotional rollercoaster may also settle down as your body starts to feel better, and you can focus on the more enjoyable aspects of pregnancy.

I am almost an inch long!

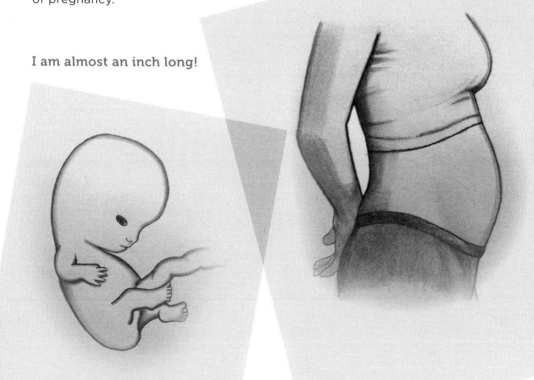

What Baby Wants You to Know

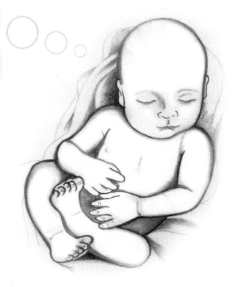

Feed me a *right*-fat, not a *low*-fat diet.

One of the best ways to gain the optimal weight for your pregnancy is to eat a "real food" diet. (See our "Healthy Pregnancy Dos and Don'ts" section for our top nutrient-dense food recommendations.)

Not only do growing baby brains need omega-3s, so do tired mommy brains! Try to eat 1,000 mg of omega-3s daily from fatty fish like salmon or supplements.

Now that you are likely beginning to feel somewhat better, and if you're up for it, exercise can be a big boost to your mood and your energy.

Bump Pic!

Date _____

Who took this picture? _____

Where was I? _____

What was on my mind? _____

_____

How was I feeling? _____

_____

What do I want to remember about this day? _____

_____

Health Check-In

Am I getting enough sleep (at least seven hours)?

_____

_____

_____

Am I staying hydrated (drinking eight or more glasses of water daily)?

_____

_____

Am I managing my stress?

_____

How?

_____

_____

Am I exercising regularly and safely?

_____

How am I doing on my healthy pregnancy goals?

_____

_____

_____

Martha's Chocolate Oatmeal Flax Bars

Nutrient-dense, homemade energy bars are a godsend when you're on the go and want to satisfy your sweet tooth in a healthy way!

1	cup butter or nonhydrogenated vegetable oil spread
1	cup honey or agave nectar
½	cup 100 percent maple syrup (or other sweetener)
2	eggs
1½	teaspoons vanilla
1¼	cups whole wheat flour
1	teaspoon baking soda
1	teaspoon salt
½	cup flaxseed meal
1	tablespoon cinnamon
½	teaspoon nutmeg
2	cups rolled oats (not instant)
12	ounces chocolate chips or carob chips (can use raisins)
	nuts or seeds, optional

Directions

Mix wet ingredients together (the first 5). Mix dry ingredients together except oats, chocolate chips, and nuts. Stir dry mixture into wet mixture. Add oats. Add chocolate chips, carob chips, or raisins, and nuts or seeds. Pour into greased glass casserole dish (the size can vary depending on how thick you want your bars). Bake at 350 degrees for about 20 minutes or until the center is cooked through. Allow to cool for at least 10 minutes before serving.

Notes

WEEK 9 What Makes Me Happy

What has been making you happy lately? What activities, foods, or environments make your body feel good? Creating awareness about what brings you joy will help you to access those happy thoughts during the rough times for a more enjoyable pregnancy.

What do I like the most about being pregnant so far?

_____

_____

_____

What are the songs I'm playing on repeat lately?

_____

_____

_____

_____

Now is a great time to start a meditation practice. Schedule a 20-minute break into your day to mellow your mind, soothe away stress, and create a daily moment of peace. Even five minutes is helpful if that is all you can spare.

What are my favorite healthy (and unhealthy) foods?

_____

_____

_____

Which physical activities am I really enjoying?

Pro-Pregnancy Tip

Take the plunge! Swimming is the ideal pregnancy exercise— it actually becomes easier while pregnant because you are more buoyant. Start a swimming routine now and, unless your health-care provider says otherwise, you can swim right up until you're ready to give birth.

What are my favorite pregnancy- and baby-related sources of information (blogs, podcasts, websites, books, magazines)?

How am I deflecting negativity in my life?

WEEK 10   Envisioning Birth . . . and What's to Come

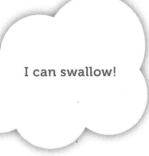

I can swallow!

Knowing there are many options for labor and birth, what are your hopes and dreams for yours? Start envisioning them now, and in the coming weeks, you'll be prompted to research and create a birth plan.

What do I want out of my birth experience?

_____

_____

_____

_____

_____

Why waste energy on things you can't change when your growing body and baby need that energy? Remember, each year millions of women go through healthy pregnancies and go on to deliver healthy babies—and many choose to do it again and again!

What are the approaches to childbirth I want to learn more about?

_____

_____

_____

_____

_____

What is shaping my idea of childbirth (movies, friends' experiences, websites . . .)?

What pregnancy and parenting resources are on my list to explore?

What are my top three concerns about when Baby comes (cost, responsibility, lack of free time . . .)?

How are my partner and I working through these concerns?

Pro-Pregnancy Tip

As you near the start of your second trimester, which is when most pregnant women feel their best, you might want to start planning a babymoon for you and your partner. Where can you go to get away, relax, and enjoy this special time in your life? Whom would you like to invite along? Make sure to check with your doctor to determine where and when are safe places and times for you to travel.

WEEK 11
Getting the Right Care for Me

Your relationship with your health-care provider is beyond important. As you begin to explore how you want to give birth (natural, medicated, water birth, or other), talk with your provider to make sure he or she is a good fit. Know that it may become necessary to switch providers to get the needed support for the type of birth you want.

What are my top five priorities for my health-care provider (for example: distance, bedside manner, experience with different birthing methods, hospital affiliation, having a midwife . . .)?

1 _____

2 _____

3 _____

4 _____

5 _____

What do I like about my current health-care provider?

_____

_____

_____

_____

_____

_____

What don't I like about my current health-care provider?

_____

_____

_____

_____

_____

What questions should I ask at my next appointment to make sure my health-care provider is a good match for me?

_____

_____

_____

_____

What pregnancy-related questions do I want to ask at my next appointment?

_____

_____

_____

_____

_____

Pro-Pregnancy Tip

Increased blood flow during pregnancy can lead to all sorts of odd symptoms, for example, bleeding gums. Swollen and bleeding gums more easily trap bacteria, which can trigger inflammation and infection elsewhere in your body. Remember to floss daily—going gentle on your gums—and go to the dentist for a check-up. Many dental plans even offer an extra cleaning during pregnancy to ensure oral health during this critical time.

WEEK 12
Keeping Up My Relationships

Now that the newness of pregnancy is wearing off, it's a good time to take a look at any areas of conflict or other issues in your close relationships. Once Baby arrives, it is too easy for this need for growth to be ignored.

How has my relationship with my partner changed over the last couple of months?

_____

_____

_____

_____

_____

What are my relationship goals? What issues do I want to address before Baby comes along?

_____

_____

_____

_____

_____

I can open and close my mouth and fists!

Try spending time with the people who lift you up and can support you during this time. Talk to your friends and family members who have already had children to help you focus on the positive aspects of your journey and all the exciting milestones you have to look forward to.

What other relationships need growth or repair, and what steps can I take in that direction?

_____

_____

_____

_____

Are there people I am hesitant to tell about my pregnancy? Who, and why?

_____

_____

_____

_____

Whom can I open up to, be honest with, and count on for support?

_____

_____

_____

_____

_____

Pro-Pregnancy Tip

If you're having a rough time adjusting to all the changes in your body and life, that's okay. Focus on what you can do for you right now and try not to worry too much about other people (if you can—this is particularly difficult if you already have kids!). Practice telling the adults in your life no. You can tell them, "I'm going through a lot right now. Don't take it personally if I'm unavailable."

Month 3 Closing Thoughts
and Final Reflections

What was the hardest part about being pregnant this month?

_____

_____

_____

_____

_____

What was the best part about being pregnant this month?

_____

_____

_____

_____

_____

When was the first time I heard Baby's heartbeat, and how did it feel?

_____

_____

_____

_____

What progress did I make on my healthy pregnancy goals?
Do I need to add to or shift my goals in any way?

What memories will I treasure from this month?

My Thoughts, Dreams, and Hopes

Use this free space to sketch, record your dreams and other random musings, or capture images, quotes, and clippings that reflect what you are feeling and focused on related to your pregnancy this month.

A Love Note (or Poem) to My Growing Baby

Dear Baby,

_____

_____

_____

_____

_____

_____

_____

_____

_____

_____

_____

_____

_____

_____

Picture of a Special Moment from Month 3!

Date _____

Who took this picture?_____

Where was I? _____

What was on my mind? _____

_____

How was I feeling? _____

_____

What do I want to remember about this day? _____

_____

Feeling Better

Weeks 13 Through 16

Congratulations! You've made it past the first trimester. For most women, the start of the second trimester is a welcome respite from the physical and emotional ups and downs of the first three months. Hopefully, that early-pregnancy exhaustion is easing up, and you're not spending so much time in bed (or in the bathroom). If so, now is the time to begin finding your new rhythm as a pregnant mama.

I'm almost 3 inches and .8 ounces!

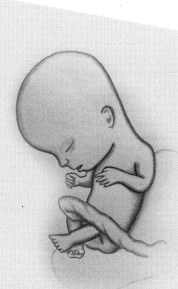

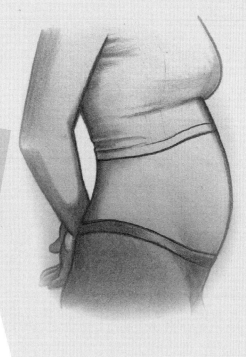

What Baby Wants You to Know

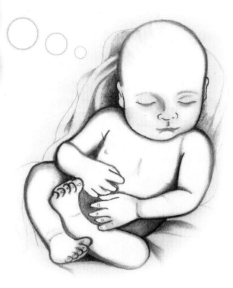

We're growing together, Mama!

Left is best. When lying down, turn to your left side to keep stomach acids down and increase the amount of blood and nutrients traveling across the placenta to me.

Graze! Try not to go too long between meals—smaller meals more often will help with any dizziness and make sure we're both well-nourished.

Don't forget your sunscreen! Pregnant mamas are especially sensitive to the sun and are prone to hyper-pigmentation.

Bump Pic!

Date _____

Who took this picture? _____

Where was I? _____

What was on my mind? _____

_____

How was I feeling? _____

_____

What do I want to remember about this day? _____

_____

Health Check-In

Am I getting enough sleep (at least seven hours)?

Am I staying hydrated (drinking eight or more glasses of water daily)?

Am I managing my stress?

How?

Am I exercising regularly and safely?

How am I doing on my healthy pregnancy goals?

Pregnancy Chicken Soup

We all know chicken soup soothes the soul, but did you know it can also soothe pregnancy discomforts, help you get the nutrients you and Baby need, and is easily digestible? Plus, it's quick to make and freeze for those inevitable times when you don't have the energy to cook.

1	large, boneless, skinless chicken breast cut into thin slices
1	egg white
¼	teaspoon salt
2	teaspoons cornstarch
¼	teaspoon white pepper
1	teaspoon sesame oil
4	cups reduced-sodium chicken broth
½	pound bok choy, cut into bite-size pieces
⅔	cup straw mushrooms
1	teaspoon sesame oil

Directions

Combine all the chicken mixture ingredients (the first 6) in a bowl and refrigerate before use. Pour the chicken broth into a 3-quart pot and bring to a rapid boil. Add the straw mushrooms and bok choy. Cook uncovered over medium heat for 2 minutes. While broth is cooking, stir in the chicken mixture. Stir to separate chicken pieces and cook briefly until chicken is done. Stir in the second teaspoon of sesame oil. Makes 4 servings.

Notes

WEEK 13 Growing along with Baby

At this stage, your regular clothing and underwear may be getting too tight, but your belly isn't big enough for maternity clothes. Buy some comfortable nonmaternity pants and skirts one size larger and with elastic waistbands. You'll wear them again after the baby is born.

What are the most noticeable changes in my body so far?

_____

_____

_____

_____

Pregnancy hormones can stimulate an increase in milky vaginal secretions that look similar to premenstrual ones. Take it as yet another sign of the changes going on in your body. On the other hand, abnormal symptoms that warrant a doctor's visit include green, yellow, cheesy, or foul-smelling secretions; burning or itching of your labia; or burning pain while urinating.

What do I love the most about my pregnant body?

_____

_____

_____

What makes me feel beautiful?

_____

_____

_____

What is my energy level? What things might be zapping
my physical and emotional energy?

_____

_____

_____

_____

Has anyone commented on my changing body?
How did it make me feel?

_____

_____

_____

_____

What are my weirdest pregnancy symptoms (cravings, food
and odor aversions, sweating, aches and pains . . .)?

_____

_____

_____

_____

Pro-Pregnancy Tip

When you are ready to
buy new, bigger bras,
think comfort above
all. Consider cotton,
which will allow
your skin to breathe.
Avoid underwire bras
because they can
compress expanding,
sensitive breast tissue.

WEEK 14   Bonding with Baby

That first sign of a bump is both exciting and a reality check as you can now visually witness the growing life inside of you.

I'm growing hair
on my head!

What's my special nickname for Baby? My partner's?

_____

_____

_____

_____

What is my favorite way to bond with Baby?

_____

_____

_____

_____

The unique relationship between you and your baby has begun. Some moms find that bonding with Baby comes naturally, and some need to be more intentional about creating this connection.

How does my partner bond with Baby?

_____

_____

_____

_____

What is the first purchase I've made, or will make, for Baby?

What are the top five things I am looking forward to about having a baby (buying cute clothes, holding Baby in my arms, taking Baby to the park, introducing Baby to my grandmother . . .)?

1 _____

2 _____

3 _____

4 _____

5 _____

If I've had an ultrasound already, what was it like to see Baby for the first time?

Pro-Pregnancy Tip

Do you feel like you have your energy back? Still, it is best to ease back slowly into your old routines. Finding your new rhythm is about exploring what works for you in this new stage. And it most likely won't mean going right back to your pre-pregnancy level of activity.

WEEK 15 Learning about Childbirth

Now is a good time to explore childbirth education. The kind of class you choose matters, and some class series start earlier in pregnancy than others. The philosophy of each method can determine how well prepared you are when the time comes.

We've listed the most common types of childbirth classes below so you can jot down your thoughts and the pros and cons of each.

International Childbirth Education Association (ICEA)

_____

_____

_____

_____

_____

The Bradley Method

_____

_____

_____

_____

_____

I can suck my thumb!

Everything is growing more rapidly during the second trimester, which equates to more weight gain for you. Nevertheless, it could still be some time before you "look pregnant" to others, especially if this is your first baby.

Hypnobirthing

_____

_____

_____

Hospital- or birthing center-based classes

_____

_____

_____

Other

_____

_____

_____

After researching all of these methods, what are my priorities for childbirth?

_____

_____

_____

_____

Childbirth Education

- The earlier you start exploring, the better. Early-bird classes offer guidance you can use throughout pregnancy.

- Bring your birthing partner with you to at least some (if not all) the class sessions.

- Classes vary widely in length—from one 3-hour class to 12 multi-hour sessions. Whatever time you choose to spend, it will be a worthwhile investment.

- Chances are, you'll find some like-minded friends there to go through pregnancy and new baby stages with!

WEEK 16
Planning My Maternity Leave

Talk to me, Mama! My hearing is starting to develop.

Before telling your employer, make sure to do your homework. Know your legal rights as well as your company's maternity leave policy. Also, consider what you want to do if your maternity leave wishes stray from your employer's policy. Determine the amount of leave you can afford and want to take and how you can work with your employer to make the transition as smooth as possible.

What does my *ideal* maternity leave and early motherhood plan look like?

_____

_____

_____

_____

Does your employer know about your pregnancy yet? The rule of thumb is to notify your work just after they begin to suspect and before they are sure—usually around 16 weeks.

What will my maternity leave and early motherhood plan *most likely* be?

_____

_____

_____

_____

Will my partner be taking any time off when Baby is born?
How can you make the most of this together time?

What kind of support is available for me after Baby is born?
Whom can I count on to help out?

If my feelings about working after Baby comes or my ability
or need to go back to work change, what are my options?

Pro-Pregnancy Tip

Breastfeeding after you go back to work can require some planning ahead. Check with your insurance provider to see if it will cover the cost of a breast pump. There may be some paperwork needed, such as a prescription from your doctor for your baby to continue to be fed breastmilk. It's better to find out all the details early on so you don't have to worry about it once Baby arrives.

Month 4 Closing Thoughts
and Final Reflections

How did I announce my pregnancy?

_____

_____

_____

_____

_____

_____

What were some of my favorite reactions?

_____

_____

_____

_____

_____

_____

What progress did I make on my healthy pregnancy goals?
Do I need to add to or shift my goals in any way?

What memories will I treasure from this month?

My Thoughts, Dreams, and Hopes

Use this free space to sketch, record your dreams and other random musings, or capture images, quotes, and clippings that reflect what you are feeling and focused on related to your pregnancy this month.

A Love Note (or Poem) to My Growing Baby

Dear Baby,

Picture of a Special Moment from Month 4!

Date _____

Who took this picture?_____

Where was I? _____

What was on my mind? _____

_____

How was I feeling? _____

_____

What do I want to remember about this day? _____

_____

Obviously Pregnant

Weeks 17 Through 20

Believe it or not, you are almost halfway there! You may find yourself often with your hand on your belly as a way to connect with or subconsciously protect your growing baby. This halfway point may also mark the best of how you've felt so far—and will feel going forward. If that's the case, embrace it! Tackle that pregnancy bucket list, take a fun vacation with your partner, and enjoy your pregnancy glow.

I'm over 5 inches and weigh 5 ounces!

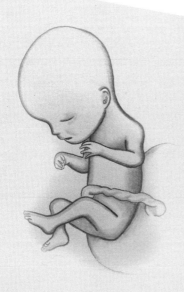

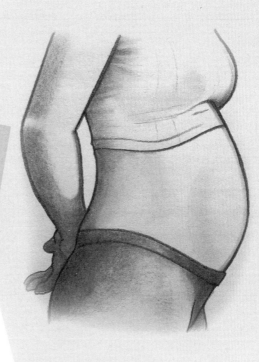

What Baby Wants You to Know

Introduce me to my family, Mama!

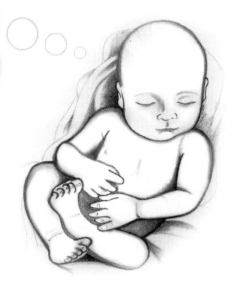

Like your skin, your eyes may be extra sensitive to light right now. Make sure to wear sunglasses that block out UVA and UVB rays whenever you're outside.

Now's a great time for me and my family members to get to know each other (siblings, cousins, aunts, grandparents, and so on). Help them to feel my little kicks and ask them to talk to me!

Time to put away the high heels! I'm big enough now to alter your posture and sense of balance so it's better to be safe.

Bump Pic!

Date _____

Who took this picture? _____

Where was I? _____

What was on my mind? _____

_____

How was I feeling? _____

_____

What do I want to remember about this day? _____

_____

Health Check-In

Am I getting enough sleep (at least seven hours)?

_____

_____

_____

Am I staying hydrated (drinking eight or more glasses of water daily)?

_____

_____

Am I managing my stress?

_____

How?

_____

_____

Am I exercising regularly and safely?

_____

How am I doing on my healthy pregnancy goals?

_____

_____

_____

Superfood Chili

This nutrient-dense, easy-to-eat meal requires less than 20 minutes hands-on time and provides 12 hefty servings—plenty to freeze for later! Top your serving with some sliced avocado for an extra dose of healthy fats.

2	chopped onions
4	garlic cloves, minced
2.5	pounds lean ground turkey
4	ounces Italian turkey sausage
4	tablespoons chili powder
2	teaspoons ground cumin
2	teaspoons paprika
¼	teaspoon ground turmeric
¼	teaspoon ground coriander
¼	teaspoon ground cardamom
2	teaspoons unsweetened cocoa powder
2	8-ounce cans tomato sauce
1–2	cans kidney beans
1–2	cans pinto beans
1	tablespoon dark molasses
2	cans low-sodium vegetable broth
2	teaspoons balsamic vinegar
1	can of beer (the alcohol evaporates during cooking)

Directions

Sauté onions and garlic. Add meat and sauté until it's no longer pink. Add remaining ingredients and bring to a boil. Feel free to spice it down if you prefer it mild. Simmer for 2 hours. The lengthy simmering brings out the full flavor of the spices in the chili.

WEEK 17   Learning about Baby

We both have
so much to learn!

Most women undergo a detailed anatomy ultrasound in their second trimester to ensure the baby is growing well and to find out the sex (if you so desire). Seeing your little one on the screen may leave you and your partner speechless as you witness the wiggly little life who has taken up residence in your belly!

How did it feel to see the baby up close during the ultrasound and hear the heartbeat?

_____

_____

_____

Am I going to find out the sex or leave it as a surprise? Why or why not?

_____

_____

_____

_____

If you're lucky, your need to urinate frequently may ease up in the second trimester as your uterus rises out of your pelvis and away from your bladder.

What are my feelings about the sex of the baby?

_____

_____

_____

What do I think Baby's personality will be like?

What do I want to expose Baby to in the womb
(music, poetry, singing, variety of flavors, sunshine . . .)?

Pro-Pregnancy Tip

For whatever reason, pregnancy can produce dreams that are more intense, vivid, disturbing, and bizarre than your nonpregnant dreams. In addition, these dreams are recalled more easily because pregnant women wake up so frequently. Consider keeping paper and a pen on your bedside table to help you capture or let go of your vivid dreams and fall back asleep more easily.

WEEK 18   My Community of Mothers

Around this point, many women begin to have intense maternal emotions not only toward their babies but toward anything remotely baby-related—whether it's tearing up at the sight of a tiny diaper or at the car insurance commercial you've seen a million times before. But even if you're not feeling particularly "motherly," it's no indication of the mom you will eventually become. Like everything else in pregnancy and parenting, each person's experience is unique.

Can you feel
me kick, Mama?

What was my mother's (or close friend's or other family member's) experience of being pregnant and giving birth?

_____

_____

_____

_____

At first, your baby's kicks will feel like light fluttering—you may even mistake them for gas! And did you know that the more often you've been pregnant, the earlier you can feel them?

What parts of their stories most resonate with me?

_____

_____

_____

_____

What do I want to do the same or differently?

_____

_____

_____

_____

_____

_____

_____

What is the most helpful pregnancy advice I've received so far?
Who was it from?

_____

_____

_____

_____

_____

_____

_____

Pro-Pregnancy Tip

As the baby growing inside of you becomes a more obvious reality, it's normal to have worries or fears about all the changes to come. In some ways, thinking through these changes and how you will manage them now will make it easier to weather the adjustments after birth. But if you feel like you're ruminating and can't get the worries out of your head, it may be time to talk through your feelings with your partner, a close friend, or a professional to get some perspective.

WEEK 19 Taking Care of Me

You are doing the most important job in the world—growing a new life—and now, everyone you meet can see that with their own eyes. Around the fifth month is when pregnant moms start getting the special treatment from strangers. Hopefully your friends and family have been treating you well all along!

How am I practicing self-care (massage, warm baths, meditation, long walks in nature . . .)?

_____

_____

_____

_____

_____

How am I feeling now compared to in the first trimester? What new rhythms am I settling into?

_____

_____

_____

_____

_____

What in my life is going better than expected?

What is the hardest thing I'm dealing with?
How am I dealing with it?

What projects are hanging over my head that I can take on
or complete that would give me a sense of accomplishment?

Pro-Pregnancy Tip

You probably know that eating for two doesn't mean eating twice as much—after all, that second person is teeny tiny in comparison to you! At this stage, eating right means adding about 300 calories of healthy protein, healthy fats, fruits, and veggies to your daily diet. Try to avoid extra desserts, sugary drinks, and other empty-calorie foods like chips. Quality is a much better goal than quantity.

WEEK 20 Healthy Habits

Itchy belly? As the skin around your hips and abdomen stretches to accommodate Baby, it is common to feel itchy. Make an anti-itch oatmeal bath by adding a half-cup of uncooked quick oatmeal to warm (not hot) bath water. An all-natural stretch-mark cream, coconut oil, or cocoa butter can also help.

I have my own unique fingerprints!

How have my eating patterns changed?

_____

_____

_____

_____

_____

While your hair and nails may be growing in longer and thicker as a side effect of pregnancy, you may find hair growing in some unwanted places as well. Shaving, electrolysis, and waxing are safe, but avoid chemical hair removers and bleaches.

What have been the hardest things for me to cut out or cut back on?

_____

_____

_____

_____

_____

How does my health-care provider feel about my weight gain so far?

Pro-Pregnancy Tip

If you're feeling up to it, see what fitness classes specifically for pregnant women your neighborhood has to offer. Trained instructors can help you learn to move in ways that support your growing body, strengthen the muscles needed for birthing, and even relieve pregnancy-related discomforts. Classes are also a great way to find moms in the same boat as you to share your pregnancy joys and woes with. But if classes aren't your thing, you can also find a plethora of prenatal fitness resources and videos online.

What was my pre-pregnancy fitness routine?
How is it different now, and what do I miss the most?

What new healthy habit am I most proud of?

What are my favorite ways to get moving? Who can I recruit
to be my workout buddy and keep me accountable?

Month 5 Closing Thoughts
and Final Reflections

Now that I am halfway through my pregnancy, I feel . . .

_____

_____

_____

_____

My most memorable pregnancy dream so far was:

_____

_____

_____

What's on my pregnancy bucket list (travel, dine at special restaurants,
go to the theater, visit friends . . .)?

_____

_____

_____

_____

What progress did I make on my healthy pregnancy goals?
Do I need to add to or shift my goals in any way?

What memories will I treasure from this month?

My Thoughts, Dreams, and Hopes

Use this free space to sketch, record your dreams and other random musings, or capture images, quotes, and clippings that reflect what you are feeling and focused on related to your pregnancy this month.

A Love Note (or Poem) to My Growing Baby

Dear Baby,

Picture of a Special Moment from Month 5!

Date _____

Who took this picture? _____

Where was I? _____

What was on my mind? _____

_____

How was I feeling? _____

_____

What do I want to remember about this day? _____

_____

Feeling Baby Move

Weeks 21 Through 24

You've sure come a long way, Mama! Now that you're in the middle of the middle trimester, how does it feel? Hopefully you're in a physical and emotional place to appreciate the journey you and your baby have been on so far and the amazing growth that has taken place. Every day, Baby makes his or her presence more and more known with kicks and hiccups!

I'm over 10 inches and 12 ounces!

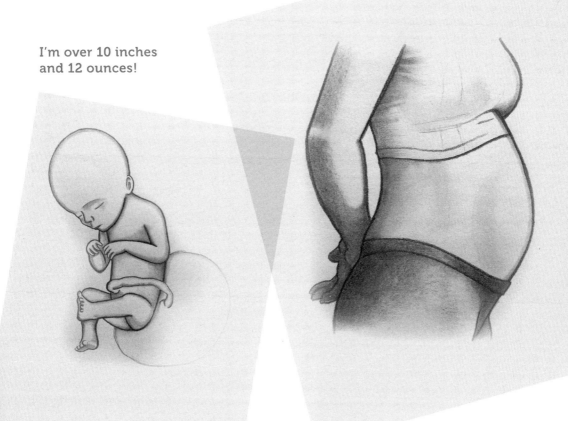

What Baby Wants You to Know

Move intentionally, Mama!

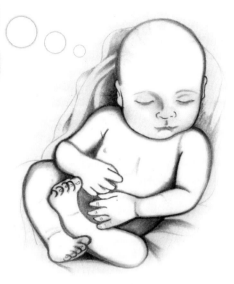

Move slowly and deliberately! Your center of gravity is gradually changing as I grow, and sudden movements could easily throw you off balance.

Lift smart! Make sure to use your legs, not your back, when lifting objects (or your toddler). Instead of bending at the waist, bend at the knees to preserve your lower back—you're going to need it for holding me.

Use your seatbelt correctly. The right way to wear a seatbelt to accommodate me is to place the lap belt as low as possible and snug across your upper thighs.

Bump Pic!

Date _____

Who took this picture? _____

Where was I? _____

What was on my mind? _____

_____

How was I feeling? _____

_____

What do I want to remember about this day? _____

_____

Health Check-In

Am I getting enough sleep (at least seven hours)?

Am I staying hydrated (drinking eight or more glasses of water daily)?

Am I managing my stress?

How?

Am I exercising regularly and safely?

How am I doing on my healthy pregnancy goals?

Healthy Pregnancy Snack: Dirty Popcorn

Make and share this easy guilt-free snack with the whole family!

organic popcorn

extra-virgin olive oil

cinnamon

sea salt

raisins (optional)

chocolate chips (optional)

Directions

Air-pop the popcorn, then put the hot popcorn into a paper bag, and add a dash of olive oil. Sprinkle with cinnamon and sea salt (or even some chocolate chips and raisins) and fold the bag closed. Shake, shake, shake, then put in a bowl, and munch away!

Notes

WEEK 21　Intimacy While Pregnant

For many women, a ramped-up sex drive comes along with a return of their energy in the second trimester. The increased blood flow and shifting hormones allow for enhanced sensation and pleasure. Unless your health-care provider says otherwise, there are no contraindications for sex during pregnancy as long as you're feeling up for it. It's also a great way to maintain the connection with your partner during this new phase of your lives together.

How does sex feel different to me now that I'm pregnant?

_____

_____

_____

How does sex feel different to my partner now that I'm pregnant?

_____

You're over halfway there, but there's still a long way to go. If you're feeling impatient, now's a good time to practice acceptance. Both pregnancies and babies move forward in their own time—might as well get used to it!

_____

_____

_____

What do I like the most about pregnancy sex?

_____

_____

_____

Have my partner and I discussed our changing sexual relationship? How did it go?

_____

_____

_____

_____

Are there other things about our relationship I want to talk with my partner about? How can I bring them up?

_____

_____

_____

_____

_____

In what other ways are my partner and I connecting that feel good?

_____

_____

_____

_____

_____

Pro-Pregnancy Tip

Mixed feelings about sex are totally normal. It may be difficult at first to appreciate your changing body, and at times, the hormonal upheaval and sick and tired feelings will press your turn-off switch. It's all normal. With the many physical and lifestyle changes that accompany becoming a parent, open and honest communication about sex with your partner remains key.

WEEK 22
Aches, Pains, and Baby Moves

I've been doing somersaults! Can you feel them?

Can you avoid standing or sitting for long periods of time? Both can promote cramping and enlarged veins during pregnancy (the dreaded varicose veins). When sitting, don't cross your legs. Instead, try to elevate your feet or do leg pumping exercises: flex and point your toes and kick your legs back and forth to increase circulation.

What was it like to feel Baby's first kicks?

_____

_____

_____

_____

Many women report heartburn relief when assuming the hands and knees position. It takes advantage of gravity to pull the uterus away from the stomach and allows the stomach contents to move more easily down into the intestines instead of refluxing up into the esophagus.

What are other people's reactions to feeling the baby kick?

_____

_____

_____

_____

_____

What does it look and feel like when Baby moves around inside me?

Which parts of my body ache the most, and how am I managing the discomfort?

What are some of my most embarrassing pregnancy moments so far (pregnancy brain, clumsiness, unexpected bodily emissions . . .)?

Pro-Pregnancy Tip

As Baby grows, so will the pressure on your lower back. Here are the best ways to minimize and relieve back pain during pregnancy:

1. Keep your head up: looking down puts extra strain on your back and neck muscles.

2. Tilt your hips: pitch your hips and pelvis forward slightly and tuck in your buttocks while standing.

3. Support your lumbar: invest in a lower back cushion to preserve the natural curve of your spine while sitting.

WEEK 23
What Mothering Means to Me

I have the hiccups! Can you feel them?

Now is a good time to explore books and resources as you start considering your parenting style and how it meshes with your partner's. Your parenting approach will likely evolve over the coming years as you get to know this child's unique temperament. Observing and talking with parents you respect is another great way to help develop your parenting philosophy with your partner.

What does "mothering" mean to me?

_____

_____

_____

_____

_____

As your breasts and belly grow, stretch marks may begin to appear. Whether you get them or not is mostly genetic, but you can reduce their appearance by keeping your skin moisturized and your body hydrated.

What are five things my mother (and/or grandmother) embodied that I want to be for my child?

1 _____

2 _____

3 _____

4 _____

5 _____

Will I be a younger mom or an older mom?
What are my thoughts and feelings about that?

_____

_____

_____

_____

_____

_____

Interview your partner to answer the questions below.

What does "parenting" mean to you? Where do we agree
and disagree?

_____

_____

_____

_____

_____

_____

What are five things your mother embodied that *you* want
for our child?

1 _____

2 _____

3 _____

4 _____

5 _____

Pro-Pregnancy Tip

Has your belly
button popped out
yet? As your uterus
rises and presses
outward beneath
your navel, your
"innie" may become
an "outie"—but only
for the rest of your
pregnancy. Once you
give birth, your belly
button will go back
to normal.

WEEK 24 New Family Rituals

Now that there's another person, family bonding through rituals becomes extra special. You may naturally or intentionally find ways to connect with Baby and bring in other family members. When you find what resonates with you, these simple rituals can help all of you enjoy the pregnancy and be more mentally and emotionally prepared for Baby's arrival.

Mama, I gained a whole pound this month!

What are the sounds that get Baby's attention?
How does Baby react?

_____

_____

_____

_____

_____

At 24 weeks, your baby may be turning his or her head in response to noises and voices on the outside. Some researchers say that Baby may also be able to sense your emotions, with your soothing voice as calming and your anxious voice as upsetting.

What are some songs, important to our family,
that I want to play for Baby in the womb?

1 _____

2 _____

3 _____

4 _____

5 _____

How are my family members connecting with Baby
(reading stories, kissing my belly, singing for Baby . . .)?

_____

_____

_____

_____

Pro-Pregnancy Tip

How are your kids
feeling about their
soon-to-come new
sibling? Get them used
to the idea by letting
them talk (and sing
and read) to Baby and
letting them put their
hands gently on your
belly to feel those
little kicks.

What family rituals did you or your partner have growing up
that you want to carry on after Baby is born?

_____

_____

_____

What are some new rituals we can use to start to bond as a
family (greeting Baby each morning and saying goodnight,
praying together, tapping belly to get Baby's attention,
including Baby in family time . . .)?

1 _____

2 _____

3 _____

4 _____

5 _____

Month 6 Closing Thoughts
and Final Reflections

What were my craziest pregnancy-related internet searches this month?

_____

_____

_____

_____

_____

_____

What progress did I make on my healthy pregnancy goals?
Do I need to add to or shift my goals in any way?

_____

_____

_____

_____

_____

_____

What are my favorite baby names so far?

NAME	ORIGIN AND MEANING

What memories will I treasure from this month?

My Thoughts, Dreams, and Hopes

Use this free space to sketch, record your dreams and other random musings, or capture images, quotes, and clippings that reflect what you are feeling and focused on related to your pregnancy this month.

A Love Note (or Poem) to My Growing Baby

Dear Baby,

Picture of a Special Moment from Month 6!

Date _____

Who took this picture? _____

Where was I? _____

What was on my mind? _____

_____

How was I feeling? _____

_____

What do I want to remember about this day? _____

_____

MONTH 7
Bigger and Loving It

Weeks 25 Through 28

You are now entering the beginning of the third trimester! As Baby's due date draws nearer, you may be motivated to check off more items on your to-do lists. Go for it, Mama! After seven months, hopefully you've become used to the quirks of this pregnancy and know what you can handle and when you need to rest. Whatever you do, keep on listening to your body and be tender with yourself. Do what you can—while you still can! But also hold space for reflection on this precious and fleeting time in your life.

I am 13.5 inches
and 1.5 pounds!

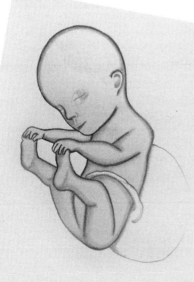

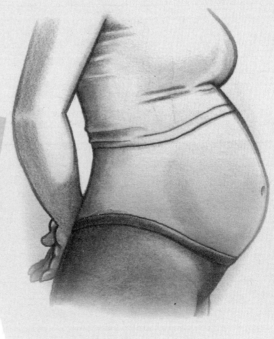

123

What Baby Wants You to Know

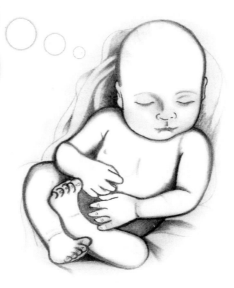

You know what they say: rest while you still can!

I feel like we are getting to know each other more and more every day.

Treat yourself! I'm getting bigger and harder to carry, I know. Help your body to relax and help relieve the aches with a soothing massage or warm soak in the bathtub when you can.

You look beautiful! Your new curves are an indication of how well you're taking care of both of us and the extraordinary mama you already are.

Bump Pic!

Date _____

Who took this picture? _____

Where was I? _____

What was on my mind? _____

_____

How was I feeling? _____

_____

What do I want to remember about this day? _____

_____

Health Check-In

Am I getting enough sleep (at least seven hours)?

_____

_____

_____

Am I staying hydrated (drinking eight or more glasses of water daily)?

_____

_____

Am I managing my stress?

_____

How?

_____

_____

Am I exercising regularly and safely?

_____

How am I doing on my healthy pregnancy goals?

_____

_____

_____

Zucchini Pancakes

This is a long-standing Sears family favorite that even our toddlers enjoyed! Top with salsa, and it's a yummy savory snack, or make it a sweet treat with the addition of a fruity spread.

1   cup (or more) shredded zucchini

1   egg

½   teaspoon baking powder

    dash of salt

1   tablespoon sunflower or
    sesame seeds (for children over four)

    fruit spread or mild salsa for topping

Directions

Stir ingredients together without overbeating.
Bake on a preheated griddle. The recipe makes one, thick, 8-inch pancake or 4 mini pancakes. Before flipping, sprinkle on sunflower or sesame seeds, if desired.

Notes

WEEK 25   Planning for Birth

While you can never know exactly how your labor will unfold, it's important to be clear on what you want to happen so that your health-care team and support team (partner, doula, mother, and so on) can help make your wishes come true to the extent possible. Your childbirth class instructor and health-care provider can help you understand your options as you consider these questions.

I love our little world!

Visualize your ideal birth: Where will it take place? Who is present? Describe the environment and how you want to feel. How much pain are you okay with? What kinds of medical interventions are acceptable to you?

_____

_____

_____

_____

_____

Now is a good time to start thinking about your birth plan and wishes. Where would you like to give birth? Are you planning on using a birth doula (labor support person)? Whom do you want in the room with you? Are you interested in pain medication? If so, which ones?

Have I decided to hire a doula? Why or why not?

_____

_____

_____

_____

_____

Whom do I want with me when I give birth, and what do I want their roles to be?

What is my greatest fear about giving birth?

How can I manage my expectations ahead of time so as not to get overly disappointed if things don't go as planned?

Pro-Pregnancy Tip

A doula is a certified labor coach who supports you throughout labor and delivery. She is there to provide emotional and physical support and also to counsel your partner (or whomever you choose to be in the room with you) on how best to be there for you. Doulas have been shown to have a positive impact on the birthing experience for the entire family, and their presence can even result in shorter labors and fewer medical interventions. That said, many insurance plans do not cover the hiring of doulas, and their fees can range from $400 to $2,000 depending on where you live.

WEEK 26 All the Feelings

The third trimester can be a time of heightened emotions. Practicing emotional resilience and giving yourself the space to feel and grow into your new roles is important. Think of ways you can be kind and gentle with yourself (and your partner) as you enter this new phase of your lives.

What am I very sensitive about currently?

_____

_____

_____

_____

_____

During this month, you may begin experiencing Braxton-Hicks contractions or "practice" contractions as your uterus starts preparing for labor. Don't worry, they don't mean that you're going to give birth anytime soon! These contractions tone your uterus for the big event and are usually not painful. Instead they may feel like a tightening across your lower abdomen and pelvic region.

What is my overall mood (happy, excited, scared, resentful, tired, frustrated . . .)? How has it been shifting over the past few months?

_____

_____

_____

_____

_____

How do I think I have grown emotionally (more patient, better able to handle stress, more lighthearted . . .)?

_____

_____

_____

_____

Which emotional skills do I want to work on before Baby arrives?

_____

_____

_____

_____

_____

List any mothering-related experiences you want to process before you give birth:

_____

_____

_____

_____

_____

Pro-Pregnancy Tip

While most of us have heard of postpartum depression, did you know that prenatal depression can also occur? Pregnancy-related depression can include feelings of panic and being overwhelmed as well as increased crying and sleeping problems due to sadness. As with any kind of mental health issue, it is best to seek out the help and support of a qualified health-care professional.

WEEK 27   Sleep, Precious Sleep

As your body works hard to deliver oxygen to you and Baby, you may find yourself more sleepy and prone to dozing off even as night sleep becomes more difficult. Here's a deep breathing exercise for a quick pick-me-up:

1. *Stand up, arms at your sides.*

2. *Slowly raise your arms upward and outward while inhaling slowly and deeply.*

3. *Lower your arms as you slowly exhale, pushing all the air out using your diaphragm.*

How tired am I on a daily basis from 1 (exhausted) to 10 (fully rested)? How can I get closer to a 10?

_____

_____

_____

_____

How have my sleep patterns evolved since becoming pregnant? How has my partner been affected?

_____

_____

_____

_____

_____

I'm starting to fatten up!

From wombmate to roommate, the latest American Academy of Pediatrics (AAP) recommendations are for Baby to sleep in the same room as Mom for at least six months, preferably the first year of life. In the meantime, your carefully designed nursery can house all of Baby's belongings and changing table.

What is my bedtime wind-down routine?

What are some of my favorite nighttime snacks?

What are my and my partner's thoughts on sharing a room with Baby? We encourage you to further research the benefits of room-sharing with Baby (see the resources section).

Pro-Pregnancy Tip

Sleeping while pregnant is not easy, what with frequent urination and a growing belly getting in the way. These tips may help you get a more restful night.

1. In the evening, eat foods that contain tryptophan, which helps promote sleep. Examples include turkey, eggs, oatmeal, nuts, and cheese.

2. Make your evening meal the lightest of your day and allow a few hours for it to digest before hitting the sack.

3. If you do need a snack right before bed, make sure it contains both healthy fats and protein.

WEEK 28 Baby-Shower Time

For many, baby showers are a highlight of pregnancy. After all, when was the last time someone threw a party for you where all of your favorite people showed up just to celebrate you and shower you with presents?

What were the highlights of my baby shower?

_____

_____

_____

_____

_____

_____

Who planned it, and who attended?

Achy back, joint pain, and swollen feet—all par for the course in the third trimester! At the very least, you will have just cause to put your feet up and give your body and mind some much-needed rest.

_____

_____

_____

_____

_____

How did it feel to have all the attention on me?

What were the most special gifts we received?

Which gift was I personally most excited about?

Pro-Pregnancy Tip

Kegel exercises are the key to strengthening your pelvic-floor muscles during pregnancy. If you've started to leak urine (the infamous "sneeze-pee")—or even if you haven't—make daily Kegels a priority. You can feel the pelvic-floor muscles you need to contract by attempting to stop your urine flow midstream. Once you're familiar with the action of stopping your flow, practice doing 10 reps four times a day when you're not going to the bathroom. Work your way up to 50 reps each time.

Month 7 Closing Thoughts and Reflections

What are my current favorite things about being pregnant?

_____

_____

_____

_____

_____

_____

What are my least favorite things?

_____

_____

_____

_____

_____

_____

What progress did I make on my healthy pregnancy goals?
Do I need to add to or shift my goals in any way?

What memories will I treasure from this month?

My Thoughts, Dreams, and Hopes

Use this free space to sketch, record your dreams and other random musings, or capture images, quotes, and clippings that reflect what you are feeling and focused on related to your pregnancy this month.

A Love Note (or Poem) to My Growing Baby

Dear Baby,

Picture of a Special Moment from Month 7!

Date _____

Who took this picture? _____

Where was I? _____

What was on my mind? _____

_____

How was I feeling? _____

_____

What do I want to remember about this day? _____

_____

Almost There

Weeks 29 Through 32

With not that many weeks left, you may be eager for your due date to get here so you can finally see that precious baby you've been growing so lovingly. On the other hand, some women begin to feel anxious that they're not yet ready for all that comes after pregnancy. Regardless, there is no way to rush or stall your body—or your baby. Take a deep breath and accept that nature will take its own course in its own time. And remember, your due date is really a date range, with most babies arriving between two weeks before and two weeks after.

I am 15 inches and 2.5 pounds!

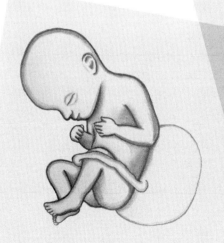

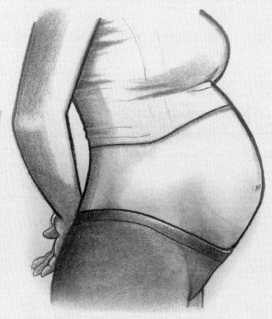

What Baby Wants to Know

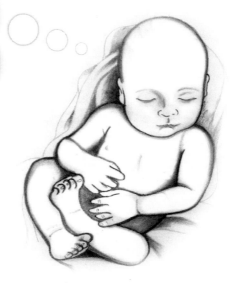

Breast milk is my favorite!

I know sleep is getting more difficult, but please still make it a priority! If seven hours of night sleep isn't happening, try for a daily catnap.

Are you researching labor pain management strategies to find the right ones for you and me?

If you are eating healthy, nutrient-dense foods, please don't stress too much about the numbers on the scale.

Bump Pic!

Date

Who took this picture?

Where was I?

What was on my mind?

How was I feeling?

What do I want to remember about this day?

Health Check-In

Am I getting enough sleep (at least seven hours)?

Am I staying hydrated (drinking eight or more glasses of water daily)?

Am I managing my stress?

How?

Am I exercising regularly and safely?

How am I doing on my healthy pregnancy goals?

Lentil Supper Soup

As Baby takes up more and more space in your body and the space for your stomach literally shrinks, soup for supper will be where it's at. This is also a great recipe to freeze and save for those newborn days when cooking will be the furthest thing from your mind.

3	tablespoons extra-virgin olive oil
3	garlic cloves, minced
2	small onions, finely chopped
1	large celery stalk, chopped
¼	cup celery leaves, chopped
½–1	pound ground turkey
2–3	carrots, thickly sliced
⅓	cup uncooked brown rice
2	tablespoons fresh parsley or cilantro, chopped
1½	cups washed lentils
1½	quarts water
1	teaspoon salt
	all-purpose natural seasoning, to taste
	black pepper, freshly ground, to taste
2	cups shredded spinach

Directions

Place lentils in a bowl and cover with cold water. Let them soak while you prepare the rest of the ingredients. Heat the oil in a large pot. Add the garlic, onion, celery, and turkey, and cook over medium heat while stirring for 5 minutes or until onions have wilted. Add the carrots, rice, parsley, and lentils. Add water and seasonings. Bring the soup to a boil. Cover it and simmer until the lentils, rice, and vegetables are tender (around 1.5 hours). Add the spinach 5 minutes before serving. Makes 4 to 5 servings.

Notes

WEEK 29   Nesting Mode

In these final months, it is common for women to want to stay close to home as well as take on household projects to prepare for Baby. You may find a sudden burst of energy and an irresistible urge to complete your home to-do list before Baby arrives. But if it gets overwhelming, don't be afraid to ask for help. Resting is just as important as nesting in month 8!

I'm enjoying my cozy nest!

In what ways have I been nesting?

_____

_____

_____

What is on my wish list of things to do around the house before Baby arrives?

_____

_____

Feeling nervous about exercise as your belly grows? Try seated exercises like chair yoga and resistance-band workouts. That way, you maintain your strength without having to worry about balance issues.

Whom am I asking and allowing to help me with everything that I want done (partner, handyman, painter, cleaner . . .)?

_____

_____

New moms like to pass on their maternity clothes. If I've received some special hand-me-downs, whom were they from?

_____

_____

_____

_____

Have I or my partner saved any special childhood items that we plan to pass down to our baby? What are they?

_____

_____

_____

_____

Where am I going to create space for Baby in our home? What will it look like?

_____

_____

_____

_____

Pro-Pregnancy Tip

Exercise remains important throughout your pregnancy, but that doesn't mean you need to be pushing yourself to the limit. If you can't maintain a conversation while exercising, then you probably need to take it down a few notches. Aim to keep your heart rate under 140 beats per minute.

WEEK 30   My Favorite Things

I'm growing
a half a pound
and a half an
inch each week!

With all the focus on the changes to your identity, both mentally and physically, it can be easy to lose track of what brings you joy. Don't put aside your favorite things. This is the time to embrace the old adage, "If Mama ain't happy, ain't nobody happy!"

What's my favorite leisure activity right now?

_____

_____

_____

_____

The pregnancy hormone relaxin is in full force toward the end of pregnancy, loosening your pelvic (and other) ligaments as your body prepares for birth. The effect may be a more pronounced waddle as you walk, as well as less stable joints that are more prone to injury. This is why it's so important to be intentional with your movements!

What is my favorite music to relax and de-stress to?

_____

_____

_____

What books am I reading or listening to for fun?

_____

_____

_____

What was the last movie(s) I saw that made me happy?

Whom do I most enjoy spending time with and why?

What is my go-to pick-me-up when I'm feeling low (time with friends, ice cream, walk in the park, cozying up on the couch with a good book . . .)?

What are my biggest sources of joy right now?

Pro-Pregnancy Tip

As your due date approaches, sleep can become more and more uncomfortable. Body pillows, leg massage, and visualization exercises can all help with relaxing your body and mind for better sleep—but they won't stop you from getting up in the middle of the night to go to the bathroom!

WEEK 31 Beautiful, Pregnant Me

The pregnant body has long been a symbol of beauty and fertility and one captured by artists throughout time. See if some of this classic art can inspire you to appreciate the beautiful, powerful goddess-in-bloom you have become.

Mama, you're my superhero!

What do I love the most about my pregnant body?

_____

_____

_____

What makes me feel beautiful?

_____

_____

_____

Around this time, Baby starts to "drop" as your body gets ready for birth. Does your bump look and feel lower yet? If not, it will likely happen soon, especially if this isn't your first pregnancy.

What are my partner's favorite things about my pregnant body?

_____

_____

_____

How have people been treating me differently now that it's so obvious I'm pregnant? How am I feeling about it?

Pro-Pregnancy Tip

As Baby gets bigger, your stomach has less room to expand. Eating smaller, more frequent meals is one of the best ways to prevent pregnancy-related reflux and indigestion.

What is the nicest compliment I've received recently? Whom was it from?

For fun, make up a superhero or goddess name for your pregnant self. In what ways do you embody this name?

WEEK 32
What Nursing Means to Me

The benefits of breastfeeding aren't just for babies! Did you know breastfeeding can help moms with postpartum recovery and weight loss, bonding with Baby, hormonal health, and reduced cancer risk?

Was I breastfed? What was my mother's experience with breastfeeding?

_____

_____

_____

_____

_____

How do I feel about breastfeeding?
What makes it attractive (or not) to me?

_____

_____

_____

_____

_____

> What's my schedule, Mama? Do I move more during the day or at night?

> Your breast milk is the perfect food for your baby as it contains the correct type and amount of fats, proteins, and carbohydrates along with a vast array of vitamins, minerals, and antibodies—the composition also changes to accommodate your baby's needs as he or she grows. The AAP recommends exclusive breastfeeding for six months, with continued breastfeeding for one year or longer, as mutually desired by mother and baby.

How does my partner feel about breastfeeding?

_____

_____

_____

_____

Where at home do I plan to feed Baby? How can I make this "nursing station" as cozy and comfortable as possible?

_____

_____

_____

_____

What advice have I received regarding breastfeeding that resonates with me?

_____

_____

_____

_____

Pro-Pregnancy Tip

If you are seeking information and support for breastfeeding, La Leche League International provides free online support and free monthly in-person gatherings with experienced leaders. Many pregnant moms have found it helpful to attend several monthly meetings to be better prepared and to start creating relationships with other new moms. La Leche League can also be an important resource if you encounter difficulties with breastfeeding. See the resources section at the back for more breastfeeding support.

Month 8 Closing Thoughts and Final Reflections

What are three highlights from my eighth month of pregnancy?

1 _____

2 _____

3 _____

What was my lowest moment?

_____

_____

_____

_____

_____

What progress did I make on my healthy pregnancy goals?
Do I need to add to or shift my goals in any way?

_____

_____

_____

_____

What are my favorite baby names so far?

NAME	ORIGIN AND MEANING

What memories will I treasure from this month?

My Thoughts, Dreams, and Hopes

Use this free space to sketch, record your dreams and other random musings, or capture images, quotes, and clippings that reflect what you are feeling and focused on related to your pregnancy this month.

A Love Note (or Poem) to My Growing Baby

Dear Baby,

Picture of a Special Moment from Month 8!

Date _____

Who took this picture? _____

Where was I? _____

What was on my mind? _____

_____

How was I feeling? _____

_____

What do I want to remember about this day? _____

_____

This Is (Almost) It

Weeks 33 Through 36

As your belly grows larger and more unwieldy, so may your excitement—and possibly impatience—over your soon-to-be new arrival. Ambivalence at this stage is also very common and so are lots of intense feelings. Ride with it all, Mama; it won't be long! And keep on listening to your body— trust that it knows exactly what you need exactly when you need it.

I am over 16 inches and weigh more than 4 pounds!

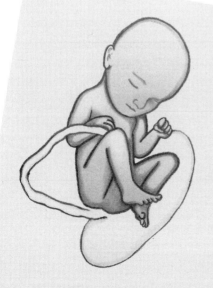

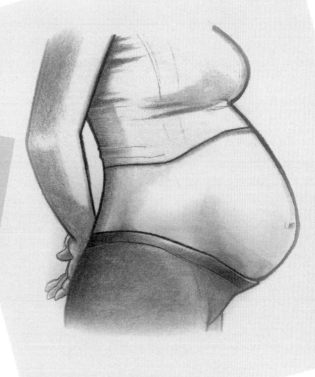

What Baby Wants You to Know

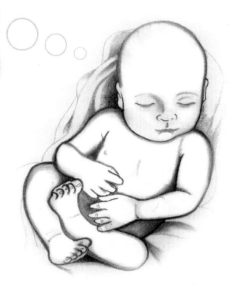

Please keep supplying me with healthy "grow" food!

After months of healthy living, it's easy to slack off toward the end. Please don't! I still need lots of healthy "grow" food, and it will help with labor and birth.

I know it's hard, but please don't slump! Good posture will help to relieve back pain and keep your muscles strong.

Explore banking my cord blood as an insurance policy for me and the rest of the family.

Bump Pic!

Date _____

Who took this picture? _____

Where was I? _____

What was on my mind? _____

_____

How was I feeling? _____

_____

What do I want to remember about this day? _____

_____

Health Check-In

Am I getting enough sleep (at least seven hours)?

Am I staying hydrated (drinking eight or more glasses of water daily)?

Am I managing my stress?

How?

Am I exercising regularly and safely?

How am I doing on my healthy pregnancy goals?

Healthy Trail Mix Recipe

This healthy trail mix is a great anytime snack of protein, carbs, and fiber to help keep your energy up, your blood sugar stable, and make sure Baby is getting all the important nutrients.

raw whole almonds

raw walnut pieces

dry-roasted, salted pumpkin seeds

dry-roasted, salted sunflower seeds

raisins

chocolate chips

your favorite "extra"

Directions

Mix all ingredients together in a bowl or bag and enjoy!

Notes

WEEK 33 Baby's Womb Personality

Baby's movements will vary according to your activity. For example, Baby will often be more still when you are moving and moving when you are still. Moms often muse about the personality of the baby based on his or her activity in the womb. After birth, you will finally see all those temperament traits in the flesh.

It's getting crowded in here!

What outside stimuli does Baby respond to (music, voices, movement, light, foods I eat . . .)?

_____

_____

_____

_____

_____

Sharp, stabbing pains around your pubic bone or at the base of your spine are, unfortunately, common in month 9. You can sometimes ease these discomforts by changing positions or with gentle exercise like yoga or long walks.

How do I experience Baby's movements when standing, walking, sitting, or lying down?

_____

_____

_____

_____

_____

When is Baby most active? What kinds of movements are most common (twists, turns, kicks, punches)?

_____

_____

_____

_____

Pro-Pregnancy Tip

Concerned that Baby hasn't moved in a while? Drink some orange juice. The extra sugar in the amniotic fluid should spur Baby into action. Try lying down on your left side to quietly count fetal kicks. At least 10 movements within two hours is considered normal.

What personality traits do I think Baby will have from me and from my partner?

_____

_____

_____

_____

What nickname has my baby bump been given lately? By whom?

_____

_____

_____

_____

WEEK 34 Bringing Baby Home

When Baby comes home, so many people will want to visit. Set boundaries for a calm and peaceful environment in which the focus is caring for and serving your needs. This is a responsibility for your partner to take on. Have your partner designate tasks like cleaning, shopping, laundry, and cooking to Baby's grandparents or other visitors. Discuss all of this with your partner beforehand and make a plan.

This is what I envision it will be like to bring Baby into our home for the first time:

_____

_____

_____

_____

_____

A favorite place for most newborns is to be held close in a baby carrier or sling. It reminds them of their time in Mama's womb and helps them feel calm and safe. Check out Babywearing International.org for more on the benefits of babywearing and choosing the right carrier.

Whom am I most excited to introduce Baby to?

_____

_____

_____

_____

_____

Whom do I want to come visit after Baby arrives, and when?
Where will they stay?

_____

_____

_____

_____

What kind of support will be the most helpful in those first
few weeks? Whom can my partner designate to do what?

_____

_____

_____

_____

_____

What are the boundaries I want my partner to enforce?

_____

_____

_____

_____

_____

Pro-Pregnancy Tip

Varicose veins, another unfortunate side effect of pregnancy, may become even more prominent in the third trimester. Ways you can reduce their appearance include eating less sodium, elevating your legs, not crossing your legs, wearing maternity-support hosiery, and drinking lots of water. On the positive side, they usually go away by the time Baby is a year old.

WEEK 35 Contingency Plans

Pain during labor is inevitable, but it doesn't have to be unbearable. Here are techniques you can practice to both lessen pain production and pain perception. A doula can support you with even more options.

- *Have a balanced mind-set about pain relief—be open to both natural and medical pain management depending on the labor experience you are having.*

- *Approach labor without fear—fear produces muscle tension and stress hormones that make labor more difficult.*

- *Play music—music you love helps occupy your mind and relax your body.*

- *Practice mental imagery and visualization—a clear mind relaxes a laboring body and encourages the production of labor-enhancing endorphins.*

- *Try laboring in water—with water supporting more of your weight, there is less muscle tension and, consequently, less pain.*

Which natural pain management strategies are the most attractive?

_____

_____

_____

_____

_____

I'm chunking up in here!

All of Baby's organs are fully developed and will function well outside the womb if he or she were born this week.

Which pain medications (if any) am I interested in getting?

_____

_____

What are my top three priorities for birth (besides a healthy baby)?

1 _____

2 _____

3 _____

How will I feel if things don't go as planned?

_____

_____

_____

How can I mentally and emotionally prepare for the unexpected?

_____

_____

_____

What preparations are we making in case I have a C-section and have to recover from major surgery right after the birth?

_____

_____

_____

Pro-Pregnancy Tip

There are times when complications make a Cesarean delivery necessary. While this may not be your first choice, it can still be a positive experience for you and Baby. Here's how:

1. An epidural anesthetic will allow you to be awake for the birth.

2. Have your partner or a loved one stay with you for support at the head of the operating table.

3. Watch as your OB lifts your baby "up and out" so you can truly witness the birth.

4. Hold your baby on your naked chest as soon after birth as possible.

5. Have your partner or loved one accompany the baby to the nursery for bonding time and your peace of mind.

WEEK 36 Final Birth Preparations

Pack your suitcase well in advance of your due date and make a practice run to the hospital or birth center to familiarize yourself with the route. It will help you determine any last-minute changes you may have to make when the moment arrives. Consider how time of day and traffic will impact your route.

What's in my hospital suitcase?
Don't forget to stash some of my favorite snacks!

_____

_____

_____

_____

What did we learn from the practice run?

_____

_____

_____

Whom do I want to notify when labor starts?

_____

_____

_____

How have my partner and I been preparing for labor?

_____

_____

_____

_____

_____

Which labor positions do I think will work best for me?

_____

_____

_____

_____

Where and how do I want to spend the majority of my time laboring?

_____

_____

_____

_____

_____

Pro-Pregnancy Tip

If you've taken a childbirth education course, you will know that lying on your back is only one of many labor positions you can try. In fact, the ones listed below will be even more effective at helping labor along:

- squatting
- kneeling
- sitting on a birthing stool or ball
- standing and leaning against your partner or a wall
- side-lying

Month 9 Closing Thoughts
and Final Reflections

What is the funniest pregnancy-related thing that happened to me?

_____

_____

_____

_____

_____

_____

Did I have any emotional freak-outs that I will laugh about one day?

_____

_____

_____

_____

_____

_____

Which of your healthy pregnancy habits do you plan on keeping?

What memories will I treasure from this month?

My Thoughts, Dreams, and Hopes

Use this free space to sketch, record your dreams and other random musings, or capture images, quotes, and clippings that reflect what you are feeling and focused on related to your pregnancy this month.

A Love Note (or Poem) to My Growing Baby

Dear Baby,

_____

_____

_____

_____

_____

_____

_____

_____

_____

_____

_____

_____

_____

_____

_____

_____

_____

_____

Picture of a Special Moment from Month 9!

Date _____

Who took this picture?_____

Where was I? _____

What was on my mind? _____

_____

How was I feeling? _____

_____

What do I want to remember about this day? _____

_____

This Is It

Weeks 37 Through 40

While it is common to think of pregnancy as being nine months, the modern way of counting the beginning of pregnancy from the first missed period makes it 40 weeks, or approximately 10 months long. Once you're in month 10, be prepared for Baby to come at any time. Most first-time moms experience their babies coming at 40 weeks (or even more!), but subsequent babies tend to make their appearance sooner—and with quicker labors to boot. This is it, Mama!

I'm over 19 inches and 6 pounds!

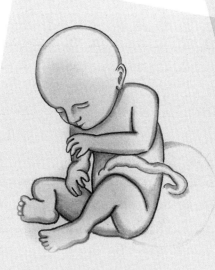

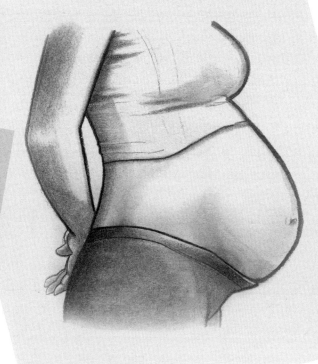

What Baby Wants You to Know

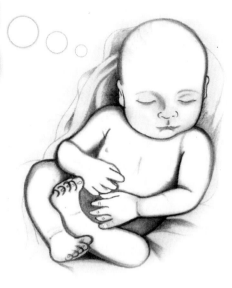

I can't wait to meet you, Mama!

Send me loving thoughts! Prenatal researchers think I can share your emotions in the womb.

A calm, soothing birthing environment will help us both have the best experience possible.

Thank you, Mama, for all that you've done for me!

Bump Pic!

Date _____

Who took this picture? _____

Where was I? _____

What was on my mind? _____

_____

How was I feeling? _____

_____

What do I want to remember about this day? _____

_____

Health Check-In

Am I getting enough sleep (at least seven hours)?

Am I staying hydrated (drinking eight or more glasses of water daily)?

Am I managing my stress?

How?

Am I exercising regularly and safely?

How am I doing on my healthy pregnancy goals?

Hearty Chicken Salad

This salad packs a lot of nutrition in a small volume and can keep in the refrigerator for a few days.

8	ounces shredded roasted chicken
2	hard-boiled eggs, chopped
¼	cup diced dill pickle
⅓–½	cup mayonnaise or Greek yogurt
1	tablespoon Dijon mustard
¼	cup sunflower seeds
1	tablespoon lemon juice
1	green onion, chopped
1	tablespoon extra-virgin olive oil
1–2	tablespoons chopped bell pepper
	salt and pepper to taste
4	whole-wheat pita pockets or tortillas

Directions

Mix the shredded chicken in a bowl with all but the last ingredient. Chill the salad and serve burrito-style on warmed whole-wheat tortillas, in a pita pocket, or add a scoop atop your green salad. For added nutrition and taste, spread a layer of hummus on the bread. Serves 2–3.

Notes

WEEK 37
Reflecting on Relationships

I can't wait to see the two of you!

Not only are pregnancy and parenthood huge life shifts, they're also likely major shifts in friendships. Friends without kids may remark that "you've disappeared." And you may notice you have less and less in common with them. Over time, many of them will catch up to this new stage of life. In the meantime, look forward to making new friends. Parenthood naturally opens up a whole new world of friendships.

How is my relationship with my partner changing?
How do I feel about it?

_____

_____

_____

Pregnancy and birth are a journey you and your partner are taking together, even though your experiences will be markedly different. In times of change, open communication is key to consider how you can grow and change together instead of apart.

How has my partner changed throughout the pregnancy?

_____

_____

_____

_____

How does my partner think I have changed?

_____

_____

_____

In what ways have I seen my friendships shifting?
How do I feel about it?

_____

_____

_____

_____

What new friends have I made so far, and how did we connect?

_____

_____

_____

_____

How can I stay connected with my nonparent friends?

_____

_____

_____

_____

Pro-Pregnancy Tip

In the last couple weeks, the mucus plug that previously sealed the cervix can be discharged. You may see anything from a teaspoonful of pink to brownish-red-tinged bloody mucous. Once you notice this "bloody show," it is possible you will go into labor soon!

WEEK 38 Being in This Body

I can grasp
things like
your finger!

As Baby drops lower into your pelvis, you may feel some relief and find it easier to breathe. Not everything gets harder the further along you are!

What have been some of my funniest "mommy brain" moments so far?

_____

_____

_____

_____

_____

_____

_____

_____

The mommy-brain struggle is real. As your due date draws near, it may feel like you are running out of brain space to remember everyday things like names, dates, and tasks. Try keeping a list of your to-dos as you think of them.

Name three things you've come to appreciate about your very pregnant body

1 _____

2 _____

3 _____

How would I describe the way my full-blown pregnant body both feels and looks?

_____

_____

_____

_____

What have been some of the hardest things to give up during pregnancy, and how have I mourned them?

Pro-Pregnancy Tip

Normal tasks—like getting up off the couch—may feel like a workout now that you're in the final stage of pregnancy. Like an endurance athlete, think through all of your movements to minimize straining and injuries.

_____

_____

_____

_____

What has gotten easier as I am reaching the end of my pregnancy?

_____

_____

_____

_____

WEEK 39 Me, Becoming a Mother

I'm getting ready to make my arrival!

Many women have mixed feelings about their pregnancy coming to an end. Ambivalence over no longer being pregnant can lead to uncertainty about making the transition from pregnancy to parenthood, especially if you are a person who doesn't handle transitions well. Realize that grieving the loss of your pregnancy is a very real need. Give yourself the time and space to deal with these late pregnancy emotions now.

What have been the biggest changes to my sense of self as I transition into motherhood?

_____

_____

_____

_____

_____

Only 1 in 10 mothers experience their bag of water breaking prior to labor. For most mothers, this doesn't happen until they are well into labor.

What do I like best about the "new" me?

_____

_____

_____

_____

_____

_____

How ready am I for this next phase of life with Baby to begin?

Pro-Pregnancy Tip

Many women, especially first-timers, can't pinpoint the exact moment active labor begins. Some of the telltale signs are regular contractions that become more frequent and intense, which start in the lower abdomen and radiate toward the back.

What parts of my pre-baby life am I most reluctant to say good-bye to?

If this is my first baby, in what ways do I already see myself as a mother?

WEEK 40 The Final Countdown

Many health-care providers request a nonstress test in this week to monitor the health of the baby. A nurse will put a belt that measures the baby's heart rate around your abdomen. All you have to do is lie back, relax, and enjoy the sound of your baby's heartbeat.

I'm full-term!

What is my biggest concern at this point (labor pains, health of Baby, C-section, being a mother, sleep deprivation, saying good-bye to my old life . . .)?

_____

_____

_____

_____

_____

What is my partner's biggest concern?

Active labor officially begins when your cervix is 4 centimeters dilated.

_____

_____

_____

_____

_____

What have I done—if anything—to induce labor naturally?

How am I feeling about sex at the moment? What other ways are my partner and I connecting physically and emotionally?

Am I ready for Baby to arrive? Or happy to have Baby inside for a while longer?

Pro-Pregnancy Tip

Baby still not here? There are many myths about how to induce labor naturally—from eating certain foods to taking a bumpy car ride. Here are some of the safest natural ways to attempt inducing labor. But remember, despite your best efforts, Baby will come when ready and not a minute before.

1. long walks

2. sexual intercourse

3. nipple stimulation

4. acupuncture and acupressure (Make sure to get your health-care provider's approval.)

5. membrane sweep to stimulate labor-starting hormones (This is done by your health-care provider.)

My Thoughts, Dreams, and Hopes

Use this free space to sketch, record your dreams and other random musings, or capture images, quotes, and clippings that reflect what you are feeling and focused on related to your pregnancy this month.

A Love Note (or Poem) to My Pre-Baby Self

What do you want to remember and cherish about who you were and how you were feeling before you gave birth?

Dear Baby,

My Baby

Baby's name

Baby's birth date and time

Baby's height and weight

A Love Note (or Poem) to My Newborn Baby

Dear Baby,

My Birth Story

My Birth Story

Picture of Baby

Date _____

Baby's age _____

Location _____

Who took this picture? _____

What do I love about it? _____

What was on my mind? _____

How was I feeling? _____

Who does Baby look like? _____

What do I want to remember about this day? _____

_____

Resources

Pregnancy, Birth, and Labor

A Child Is Born, by Lennart Nilsson (Jonathan Cape, 5th edition, 2010)

> This groundbreaking book of fetal photography from one of the world's leading medical and scientific photographers takes you on a photographic journey from fertilization to delivery.

Childbirth Without Fear: The Principles and Practice of Natural Childbirth, by Grantly Dick-Read (Pinter and Martin, 2013)

> This essential reading helps mothers ease their fear and anxiety regarding childbirth.

The Healthy Pregnancy Book: Everything You Need to Know from America's Baby Experts!, by William Sears and Martha Sears, with Linda Holt and BJ Snell (Little, Brown and Company, 2013)

> This month-by-month guide is for expectant mothers and fathers through all stages of pregnancy from preconception through birth and focuses on how to enhance the health of Mother and Baby.

The Birth Book: Everything You Need to Know to Have a Safe and Satisfying Birth, by William Sears and Martha Sears (Little, Brown and Company, 1999)

> This book provides vital advice on the events leading up to and surrounding birth and a collection of wide-ranging birth stories to put soon-to-be parents at ease.

Doulas of North America International, dona.org

> The leading doula certifying organization, this nonprofit provides a database to help you find the right labor support person for you in your area.

Parenting

The Baby Book: Everything You Need to Know about Your Baby—From Birth to Age Two, by William Sears, Martha Sears, Robert Sears, and James Sears (Little, Brown and Company, revised edition, 2013)

> This useful companion to *The Healthy Pregnancy Book* was written to help get new parents off to the right start with their newborns.

The Portable Pediatrician: Everything You Need to Know about Your Child's Health, by William Sears, Martha Sears, Robert Sears, and James Sears (Little, Brown and Company, 2011)

> This book provides invaluable information on common childhood illnesses and emergencies, including when to call the doctor, reassuring signs that your child is okay, and how to treat your child at home—all in a convenient A-to-Z format.

Baby on the Way, by William Sears, Martha Sears, and Christie Watts Kelly (Little, Brown and Company, 2001)

> A precious picture book introduces older siblings to Baby during pregnancy.

Becoming a Father: How to Nurture and Enjoy Your Family, The Growing Family Series, by William Sears (La Leche League International, 2003)

> This book offers a collection of Dr. Bill's fathering tips on being the best dad you can be.

25 Things Every New Dad Should Know: Essential First Steps for Fathers, by Robert W. Sears and James M. Sears (Harvard Common Press, 2017)

> After birth, most of the attention is (rightly) on Baby and Mama. This book shows new dads what to expect so they can support their families and get the most out of the amazing newborn journey.

25 Things Every New Mom Should Know: Essential First Steps for Mothers, by Martha Sears with William Sears (Harvard Common Press, 2017)

> Some things about mothering come naturally; others do not. This book offers insightful tips and helps new moms gain perspective as they transition into their new roles.

The Baby Sleep Book: The Complete Guide to a Good Night's Rest for the Whole Family, by William Sears, Robert Sears, James Sears, and Martha Sears (Little, Brown, and Company, 2005)

> This resource explains how to create a sleep plan that suits the needs of the entire family, giving a flexible and sensitive approach to solving babies' sleep problems rather than a one-method-fits-all approach.

Attachment Parenting International (API), attachmentparenting.org

> This network of experienced parents offers essential tools, resources, and support groups for those interested in the attachment parenting philosophy.

Postpartum Depression Facts, National Institute of Mental Health

> As a new parent, it may be difficult to know if what you're feeling is sleep deprivation, baby blues, or actual postpartum depression. Read more on postpartum depression and what to do if you think you have it at nimh.nih.gov/health/publications/postpartum-depressionfacts/index.shtml.

Babywearing International, babywearinginternational.org

> This nonprofit provides free educational meetings to help you find the best carrier for your baby and lifestyle.

Balboa Baby, balboababy.com

> This website contains a collection of Dr. Sears–designed baby carriers, nursing pillows, and other helpful items that make life cozier for babies—and easier for parents.

Arm's Reach Co-Sleeper, armsreach.com

> This bedside bassinet enables Baby and Mother to safely sleep close to each other for easier nighttime comforting and feeding.

Breastfeeding

The Breastfeeding Book, by Martha Sears and William Sears (Little, Brown and Company, 2018)

> This book contains everything you need to know about nursing your child from birth through weaning.

La Leche League International (LLLI), lalecheleague.org

> This is the most experienced and trusted resource and support group for breastfeeding mothers.

Nutrition

L.E.A.N. Expectations, drsearswellnessinstitute.org

A resource for online interactive workshops that teach expectant mothers the best health and nutrition habits for their family's well-being.

The Family Nutrition Book, by William Sears (Little, Brown and Company, 1999)

This book offers everything you need to know about feeding your children from birth through adolescence.

Juice Plus+ Whole Food Nutrition, sears.juiceplus.com

An online store for concentrated fruits, vegetables, and berries in a capsule and complete whole food–based protein shake mix.

The Authors

Martha Sears

Martha is a registered nurse, former childbirth educator, La Leche League leader, and lactation consultant. With renowned pediatrician William Sears, Martha is the coauthor of more than 25 parenting books, drawing on her experience with their eight children (including Stephen, who has Down syndrome, and Lauren, their adopted daughter). She contributes to the content of AskDrSears.com and is noted for her advice on how to handle the most common problems facing today's mothers with their changing lifestyles. Martha lives in Southern California and is blessed to spend tons of time with her grandchildren. She enjoys reading, gardening, sailing, and ballroom dancing with her husband of 53 years.

Hayden Sears

Hayden Sears, mother of three, is a certified health and nutrition coach who loves helping families and individuals on their journey toward better health. The oldest daughter of Dr. William and Martha Sears, she has worked with the Sears Family Pediatrics medical practice for over 15 years as Wellness Coordinator. She also contributes to the content of AskDrSears.com; has been a guest on TV shows and news stations sharing nutrition tips, healthy meal options, and the benefits of babywearing; and is excited to co-host the Dr. Sears Family Podcast. Hayden owns a Juice Plus+ virtual franchise and travels all over the world speaking about how to keep moms and families healthy. She received her master's degree from Azusa Pacific University and resides in Southern California. Having homeschooled for 10 years, she now volunteers at her kids' schools and enjoys dancing, performing arts, and yoga.

ABOUT
Sounds True

Sounds True is a multimedia publisher whose mission is to inspire and support personal transformation and spiritual awakening. Founded in 1985 and located in Boulder, Colorado, we work with many of the leading spiritual teachers, thinkers, healers, and visionary artists of our time. We strive with every title to preserve the essential "living wisdom" of the author or artist. It is our goal to create products that not only provide information to a reader or listener, but that also embody the quality of a wisdom transmission.

For those seeking genuine transformation, Sounds True is your trusted partner. At SoundsTrue.com you will find a wealth of free resources to support your journey, including exclusive weekly audio interviews, free downloads, interactive learning tools, and other special savings on all our titles.

To learn more, please visit SoundsTrue.com/freegifts or call us toll-free at 800.333.9185.

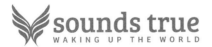